Contents

About the authors

Andrew J Pollard is Senior Lecturer in Paediatric Infectious Diseases at the University of Oxford and an Honorary Consultant Paediatrician at the John Radcliffe Hospital, Oxford, UK. He is the consultant in charge of the Oxford Vaccine Group, based in the Oxford University Centre for Clinical Vaccinology and Tropical Medicine. He is also the editor of a textbook on meningococcal vaccines, a travel medicine handbook (also with DRM), a guide for parents of children with meningitis, and over 100 medical and scientific articles. He began climbing as a medical student, and has made first British ascents of Janoli (6632 m), Garhwal, India in 1988 and Chamlang (7319 m), Eastern Nepal in 1991. He reached 8600 m on Mount Everest as the deputy leader of the 1994 British Mount Everest Medical Expedition. He is a member of the Alpine Club, a previous Editor of the Newsletter of the International Society for Mountain Medicine and a member of the editorial board of *High Altitude Medicine and Biology*. He continues to be involved in research and education about mountain and high altitude medicine, and founded a series of courses on the subject in 1993 that continues a decade later.

David R Murdoch is Professor of Pathology, Clinical Microbiologist and Infectious Diseases Physician in Christchurch, New Zealand and Adjunct Assistant Professor in Medicine at Duke University, USA. He has been spending time in the mountains since his early school days, and has since climbed and trekked in the Himalaya and Europe, as well as in New Zealand. He spent over two years working in the Mount Everest region of Nepal, first at the Himalayan Rescue Association's high altitude aid post at Pheriche, and then at Kunde Hospital. He is a member of the International Society for Mountain Medicine, an honorary life member of the Himalayan Rescue Association, and a member of the editorial board of *High Altitude Medicine and Biology*.

To Rachel and Lynley, Jim, Tess, Hannah and Alex
In memory of all
those who have lost their lives on mountains

Contributors

Remote dentistry

David Geddes BDS
St Mary's
9 Kingmeadows Gardens
Peebles EH45 9LA
UK

Medico–legal considerations for treks and expeditions

Alistair Duff (Partner)
Henderson Boyd Jackson WS
Edinburgh EH3 8EH
UK

Children's Lake Louise Acute Mountain Sickness Score

Susan Niermeyer MD (Associate Professor of Pediatrics)
Michael Yaron MD (Associate Professor of Surgery)
University of Colorado School of Medicine
Denver
Colorado
USA

Foreword by
Sir Edmund Hillary

I was 33 years old when I climbed Mount Everest in 1953 and there was no doubt that at that stage of my life I acclimatized to altitude very readily. I could run freely up the Tengboche hill at 3900 m and even above 6000 m I experienced little shortage of breath and have no recollection of suffering from periodic breathing. My main problems at extreme altitude were difficulty in sleeping well and a considerable disinterest in food. At our highest camp at 8454 m we spent 16 hours working and resting but only slept comfortably for the four hours when we were breathing oxygen at the low rate of 1 litre a minute. And yet during the other 12 hours we were able to work slowly but effectively without oxygen and suffered little discomfort. For the twenty minutes we remained on the summit of Mount Everest I removed my oxygen equipment in order to take photographs down all the leading ridges of the mountain and the film turned out particularly well, even though our physiologists had warned us that the removal of our oxygen on the top of Mount Everest might well prove disastrous. Of course, as we now know, quite a number of people have been successful in reaching the summit of Mount Everest without using oxygen. But it is still a somewhat marginal experience.

To my surprise, as the years passed, I became increasingly affected by altitude. The last two times, in 1977 and 1980, I slept for several days above 5200 m. I suffered in both cases from cerebral oedema and had to be hastily conducted down to lower levels. As I reach my late seventies I find I can only sleep comfortably below 3000 m, although I can still helicopter easily to over 4000 m and spend six or eight hours there with no difficulties apart from a certain shortage of breath and some slowness of movement. My many medical friends who specialize in high altitude physiology have difficulty in explaining my symptoms.

And this is the problem with altitude. Its effects are frequently very unpredictable.

A great deal of research has been undertaken into the problems associated with acute mountain sickness, but it is still extremely difficult to forecast who is likely to be struck down by it. It can happen equally to the young or the elderly, to the fit or the not so fit, to the experienced or the completely inexperienced. But the symptoms are very much the same in every case: headaches and nausea, vomiting and a vast feeling of lassitude. The greatest danger does not seem to occur when you are briefly climbing or flying to high altitudes, but much more commonly when you are sleeping for some days at more moderate heights. Although the medical experts cannot always explain the causes of acute mountain sickness, they can recommend procedures that should be followed if a trekker or climber shows any of the symptoms. To carry on higher either in a spirit of competitiveness or in shame at being regarded as a weaker member of your party can only in most cases aggravate the condition and even result quite rapidly in death, whereas sensible care, including a short period at lower altitudes, can overcome the problem and often enables you to recover sufficiently to make a successful effort to reach your altitude objective.

David Murdoch spent two years working at Kunde Hospital at an altitude of 3850 m, and has wide experience of dealing with people suffering from high altitude problems. Andrew Pollard has also taken part in many Himalayan expeditions and has studied and treated many people who have experienced major altitude difficulties. Their book not only discusses the technical changes that take place at altitude, but also gives sound information on how the difficulties can be sensibly handled. It is valuable reading not only for expedition medical staff, but for any who venture into the thin air of the world's highest mountains.

Sir Edmund Hillary
August 1996

Foreword by
Dr Robert B Schoene

The Third Edition of *The High Altitude Medicine Handbook* is a marvelous example of 'the fellowship of the rope' – the oft-used metaphor for individuals with a passion, coming together as a team with an unspoken commitment to a common goal, undertaken for the right reasons and carried out with the right staff. Andy Pollard and David Murdoch are two such individuals whose forays into the mountains and medicine many years ago serendipitously led them eventually to each other. Their friendship and combined energies resulted in the Handbook, now embarking on its third edition.

To understand better the genesis of the book, I asked Andy and David how they were lured to the mountains and how they got together. As suspected, their stories were not much different from my own.

Andy, like I, was seduced by the mountains as a medical student, a particularly vulnerable time in one's life when dreams of high peaks provide sustenance for the endurance required by medical studies. Also, it usually takes an individual or two to catalyze, condone, or facilitate these somewhat unconventional activities. So it was for Andy, who came in contact with the peripatetic Dr Charlie Clarke, whose keen enthusiasm for adventure is legendary. Thus, there was not only a precedent for combining medicine and high altitude but also someone to 'rope up with'. As student chairman of the Barts (St Bartholomew's Hospital) Alpine Club, Andy received a call from Chuck Evans (son of Sir Charles Evans) to help him put together an expedition to Jaonli in the Indian Himalaya, and on a subsequent trip to the Hongu Basin over the Mera La (ironically the area of my first trip to Nepal in 1976), he encountered a trekker with HACE. The encounter was the stimulus for the Plas Y Brenin mountain medicine conference that Andy (and later Peter Barry) has run very successfully for 10 years or more.

David's affair with the mountains was in some ways more natural in that it came at an earlier age as he grew up in New Zealand with the mountains as a stage from primary school on, where hiking and climbing are an integral part of a New Zealander's upbringing. Most feel a nomadic urge, and for David the European Alps and the Himalaya followed. David, too, had a mentor in Ed Hillary, and subsequent trips to the Khumbu, first as a medical student in 1984, and then to Pheriche and the Kunde Hospital, cemented his involvement with Nepal. Medicine, travel, international health, and mountains became tight strands in the fabric of his personal and professional lives.

As they followed separate ventures, a common friend, Simon Currin, and a vigorous discussion over a high altitude medical matter, eventually tied Andy and David together as friends and collaborators on the successful Handbook which occupies an important and essential niche in the world of high altitude medicine. It is not a ponderous scientific volume that would be a better doorstop or paperweight, nor is it a light offering for the day-trekker. It is a thoughtful, useful medical text that is informative and portable which is seasoned to perfect taste with scholarly documentation and citations congruent with their backgrounds as adventurers, clinicians, and academic infectious disease specialists. In other words, it is 'just right'. As in any successful pairing or expedition, it takes two committed friends who have each other on belay, and this fine book is a tribute to that 'fellowship of the rope'.

Robert 'Brownie' Schoene MD
Seattle, Washington
USA
July 2003

Preface to the first edition

More and more people are travelling to high altitude areas of the world. The promotion of high altitude destinations by the tourism industry has resulted in easy and rapid access to these places by both the experienced and the inexperienced, the unfit and the unprepared. Many high altitude travellers have their journeys disrupted by altitude related illnesses that are often preventable; a significant number die needlessly. Despite a considerable expansion in our understanding of altitude illness, people continue to ascend too rapidly, fail to recognize the significance of symptoms and delay descent. As many altitude related illnesses are both potentially fatal and readily preventable, educating travellers about the potential health hazards at high altitude is essential. Unfortunately, information on high altitude medicine is often not readily available.

This handbook has been designed for medical practitioners, travel medicine specialists, expedition doctors and other professionals who give health advice to travellers. The comprehensive glossary should make the information contained in the book accessible to non-medical readers as well, and we have provided a fact sheet for altitude illness, written in layman's terms, which doctors might like to distribute to those who may be exposed. Our aim has been to provide practical information on medical problems encountered at high altitude in a form that can be referred to quickly. We hope the book will have a place both in the doctor's surgery and in the rucksack on a trek or expedition. However, it is not a comprehensive review, and we have purposely avoided detailed discussions about pathophysiology. With some more general topics, such as trauma and first aid, we have concentrated on areas that are important or peculiar to mountain environments. For more detailed information on these subjects, specialized textbooks should be consulted. The further reading list at the end of each chapter contains references that cover each topic, and we have included additional recommended reading at the end of the book. Some areas are controversial, and we have attempted to present a balanced view from the literature, complemented by our own experiences. For some areas, where there is a paucity of scientific data, we have presented the information as it currently stands.

For all those venturing into the high and remote mountain wildernesses of the world, we hope that this handbook will go a little way to facilitating the safe enjoyment of some of the world's most beautiful places.

Andrew J Pollard
David R Murdoch
August 1996

Preface to the third edition

The High Altitude Medicine Handbook has proved so popular that both the first and second editions (published in 1997 and 1998, respectively) and the micro-edition of the text published by Radcliffe Medical Press were out of print by early 2002. It is with pleasure that we note that the third edition of our book is being published in the year of the 50th anniversary of the first ascent of Mount Everest and the 25th anniversary of the first oxygenless ascent of the highest place on earth. An unauthorized version, printed in India (1998) and based on the first edition, has sold many copies, perhaps more than the official versions. The original text was also translated into German (published in 1998) and is available from Ullstein Mosby. In the second edition we updated and revised the text and undertook an extensive revision of the referencing of the book to make the background literature more immediately accessible. We also revised the section on hypothermia and added a section on the management of avalanche casualties. In this third edition we have updated all of the chapters to include changes in knowledge of high altitude medicine that have arisen during the five years since the second edition was published. There are more than 200 changes in the third edition. As before, in the appendices we have included a fact sheet for doctors, and our fact sheet on altitude illness for patients, which is not bound by copyright, has been converted to an algorithm with the assistance of David Hillebrandt. In producing the third edition we are grateful for comments from reviewers of the first and second editions in the medical and lay press, and especially for advice from David Hillebrandt. As before, we are very grateful for the expertise provided in the contributions of David Geddes, Alistair Duff, Michael Yaron and Susan Niermeyer.

Andrew J Pollard
David R Murdoch
July 2003

Acknowledgements

The authors are indebted to their colleagues who contributed to 'Mountain and High Altitude Medicine', a course for doctors that has been held since 1993 (and is still running in 2003) at the National Mountain Centre, Plas Y Brenin, North Wales, and also to the members of the 1994 British Mount Everest Medical Expedition, led by Dr Simon Currin, who inspired this text. We are very grateful for the contribution on remote dentistry from David Geddes, and to Alistair Duff who provided the medico–legal discussion in Chapter 11. We are hugely in debt to Dr Michael Yaron and Dr Susan Niermeyer, who provided the text for the Children's Lake Louise Score in Appendix 2. We are also grateful to Peter Pollard of the Scottish Environmental Protection Agency for help with the environmental discussion. In addition, we would like to thank Dr Nick Mason for providing the data relating altitude to oxygen saturation, Dr Richard Price for providing the chest X-ray and Dr Diana Depla for the retinal photograph. Medical Expeditions (formerly known as 'Everest Medical Expedition 1994' – a charitable company), through support of the courses mentioned above and production of the first edition of this book, has made publication possible. The authors would also like to acknowledge Professor John West, Editor of *High Altitude Medicine and Biology*, for permission to use material from the journal in Chapter 4. AJP owes a great debt to Dr Charles Clarke, who encouraged his interest in high altitude medicine as a medical student. We are also indebted to the following who helped with their comments and criticisms of the manuscript: Dr James Milledge, Dr Simon Currin, Dr Rachel Pollard, Dr Peter White, Dr Gill White, Dr David Hillebrandt, Dr Andrew Knight, Dr Carolyn Knight, Dr Peter Barry, Dr Helen Eglitis, Dr David Collier, Dr Catherine Collier, Dr Diana Depla, Dr Lynley Cook, Dr Chris Curry, Dr Jan Arnold,

Professor Peter Bärtsch, Dr Tom Egnot, Dr James Litch and Dr Evan Lloyd. In particular we wish to thank our families, who cheerfully tolerated the production of this book.

Colour plates list

1 Snowblindness. A sherpa with conjunctivitis and lid oedema following glacier travel without goggles. (L Cook)

2 Frostbite. Hands of a Tibetan refugee showing a line of demarcation between necrotic (black) and viable tissue four weeks after freezing injury. (L Cook)

3 Superficial frostbite of a climber's ankle showing blister formation. Complete healing occurred. The cold injury was associated with a fracture of the ankle caused by a fall. (D Murdoch)

4 Retinal photograph at 5300 m of a climber who later reached the summit of Everest showing vascular engorgement, tortuosity and retinal haemorrhage. (D Depla)

5 A sick climber with high altitude cerebral oedema being carried by a sherpa. (L Cook)

6 Sherpa boy in the Khumbu valley. (A Pollard)

7 River crossing. (A Pollard)

8 Postero-anterior and lateral chest radiograph showing typical appearance of HAPE. (R Price)

9 Research at Everest Base Camp on the 1994 British Mount Everest Medical Expedition. (A Pollard)

10 The Gamow portable hyperbaric tent. Note this is larger than the more commonly used 'one-person' chamber. (D Murdoch)

Introduction

High places

The main destinations where climbers, trekkers and skiers are likely to travel and put themselves at risk from high altitude illness are the Himalaya (India and Nepal), the Karakoram Mountains (Pakistan), Mount Kenya and Kilimanjaro (East Africa), the Andes (Ecuador, Peru, Bolivia, Argentina and Chile), the Rocky Mountains (North America) and the European Alps (*see* Figure 1.1). Other less recognized high altitude areas include parts of Hawaii, the Canary Islands, New Guinea, Japan, New Zealand and Antarctica.

Definition of high altitude

The concept of 'high altitude' is an arbitrary one. In lay terms it can mean anything above the height of many Alpine winter resorts at around 1500 m. In medical literature the term is more defined and based on alterations in human physiology. In this book, the term 'high altitude' can be taken to mean heights above 2500 m.

Intermediate altitude (1500–2500 m)

Physiological changes due to hypobaric hypoxia are detectable, but arterial oxygen saturation remains above 90% (*see* Figure 1.2). Altitude illness is possible.

High altitude (2500–3500 m)

Altitude illness is common with rapid ascent to above 2500 m.

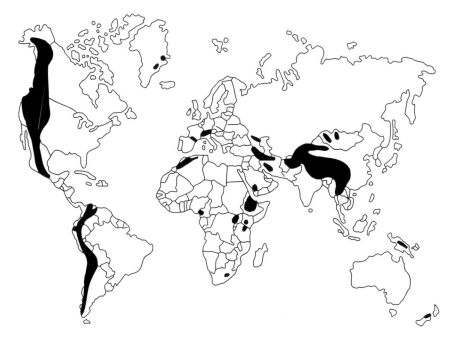

Figure 1.1: Map showing the major high altitude regions of the world apart from Antarctica.

Very high altitude (3500–5800 m)

Arterial oxygen saturation falls below 90%. Altitude illness is common and marked hypoxaemia can occur during exercise.

Extreme altitude (> 5800 m)

Further successful acclimatization cannot be achieved, progressive deterioration occurs and survival cannot be maintained permanently. Marked hypoxaemia occurs at rest.

Barometric pressure and altitude

At increasing altitudes above sea level, barometric pressure decreases and with it the partial pressure of oxygen falls (*see* Appendix 5). At the

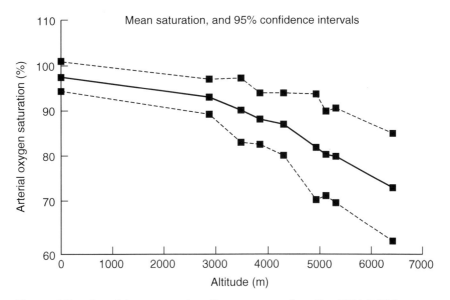

Figure 1.2: Arterial oxygen saturations measured on the 1994 British Mount Everest Medical Expedition at various altitudes (sea level, *n*=20; 2855 m, *n*=41; 3460 m, *n*=42; 3835 m, *n*=40; 4270 m, *n*=41; 4930 m, *n*=42; 5118 m, *n*=38; 5300 m, *n*=20; 6400 m, *n*=8). Data provided by Dr Nick Mason.

summit of Mont Blanc (4807 m), the highest mountain in Western Europe, the partial pressure of oxygen is about half of that at sea level, and on the summit of Mount Everest (8848 m) it is one-third of sea level pressure (*see* Figure 1.3). For a given altitude, barometric pressure is higher at the equator than at the poles, and is higher in summer than in winter.

For climbers and trekkers at altitudes above 2500 m, the lack of oxygen may cause illness that is potentially life-threatening. With the rising influx of tourists to altitude in recent years, the prevention and management of altitude induced illness has become of increasing importance to trekkers, skiers, expedition doctors, general practitioners and travel medicine specialists. In 2001 it was estimated that approximately 140 million people were living permanently at altitudes over 2500 m worldwide (Niermeyer *et al.*, 2001), and nearly the same number of low altitude sojourners are visiting these areas annually (Moore, 1987). The number of high altitude visitors has certainly increased since. Around one million people travel to developing countries from the UK each year, and up to 50% will become

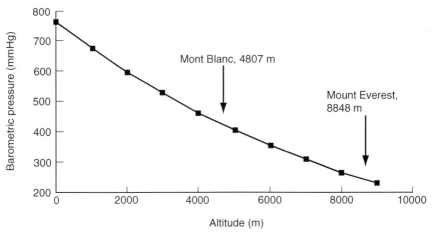

Barometric pressure falls as altitude increases

Figure 1.3: Change in barometric pressure with altitude.

unwell during or after their trip (McIntosh, 1993). Health advice before travel may prevent many of these illnesses.

In Nepal, although there were some 100 000 visitors (20 000 from the UK) to altitude in 1991, less than 1% were registered as members of a mountaineering expedition by the Ministry of Tourism. Although trekkers are the largest group exposed to high altitude, the greatest mortality occurs in climbers who expose themselves to extreme altitude. On British expeditions to peaks over 7000 m between 1968 and 1988, there was a 4.3% mortality (Pollard and Clarke, 1988). Most deaths were not directly caused by altitude illness, but were due to injuries sustained in falls or as a result of rockfall or avalanche. Many may have been attributable to disorientation and misjudgement induced by altitude hypoxia. The mortality of trekkers in Nepal is about 14 per 100 000, with 25% of these deaths being attributed to altitude illness (Shlim and Gallie, 1992).

Acclimatization

Acclimatization is the process by which individuals gradually adjust to altitude hypoxia. It is a poorly understood physiological process involving a series of adjustments that occur over a period of hours to months. These changes all favour increased oxygen delivery to cells and efficiency of oxygen use. In contrast, the term 'altitude adaptation' describes physiological changes that occur over decades and generations that confer advantages for life at altitude.

The most important component of acclimatization is an increase in ventilation (i.e. increased rate and depth of respiration). This begins to occur at altitudes of about 1500 m. With increased ventilation come hypocapnia and respiratory alkalosis, which limit further increased ventilation. As acclimatization proceeds, there is gradual renal compensation by excretion of bicarbonate that tends to restore arterial pH to near normal values. Heart rate increases with ascent although, with acclimatization, resting heart rate approaches sea-level values (except at extreme altitude). At extreme altitude, resting and maximum heart rates converge as the limits of acclimatization are approached. Erythropoietin secretion in response to hypoxaemia stimulates the production of red blood cells, resulting in increased haematocrit and haemoglobin concentrations. This response is not necessarily beneficial, as excessive polycythaemia may impair oxygen transport due to increased blood viscosity.

There is considerable individual variation in the ability to acclimatize to altitude. Some people acclimatize rapidly, while others develop acute mountain sickness and require longer periods of time to acclimatize fully. Very few people are incapable of acclimatization; virtually everyone is able to acclimatize, given sufficient time. The tendency to acclimatize rapidly or slowly is consistent on repeated altitude exposures. If someone is a 'slow acclimatizer' on one journey, the same pattern should be expected to occur on subsequent journeys to similar elevations. Although attempts to prepare for ascent by breathing hypoxic gas mixtures at sea level are impractical and are flawed by rapid loss of acclimatization (Benoit et al., 1992), periods spent in a hypobaric chamber prior to rapid ascent to high altitude may assist acclimatization (Richalet et al., 1992).

Successful acclimatization is characterized by the absence of altitude illness and improved sleep. It is relatively short-lived following descent to low altitude, with effects lasting at least eight days (Lyons et al., 1995).

Acclimatization in adults seems to be possible up to about 5000–5500 m. Above this elevation there is a fine balance between adjustment to altitude and deterioration as a result of chronic hypoxia. At more extreme altitude, deterioration becomes increasingly prominent, and above 8000 m no acclimatization occurs and prolonged exposure is incompatible with survival.

References and further reading

Benoit H, Germain M, Barthélémy JC *et al.* (1992) Pre-acclimatization to high altitude using exercise with normobaric hypoxic gas mixture. *Int J Sports Med.* **13(Suppl.)**: S213–16.

Lyons TP, Muza SR, Rock PB *et al.* (1995) The effect of altitude pre-acclimatization on acute mountain sickness during re-exposure. *Aviat Space Environ Med.* **65**: 957–62.

McIntosh IB (1993) Introduction. In: IB Mcintosh (ed.) *Health, Hazard and the Higher-Risk Traveller*. Quay Publishing, Lancaster, pp. vii–xix.

Moore LG (1987) Altitude-aggravated illness: examples from pregnancy and prenatal life. *Ann Emerg Med.* **16**: 965–73.

Niermeyer S, Zamudio S and Moore LG (2001) The people. In: TF Hornbein and RB Schoene (eds) *High Altitude: an exploration of human adaptation*. Marcel Dekker Inc., New York, pp. 43–100.

Pollard A and Clarke C (1988) Deaths during mountaineering at extreme altitude. *Lancet.* **i**: 1277.

Richalet J-P, Bittel J, Herry J-P *et al.* (1992) Pre-acclimatization to high altitude in a hypobaric chamber: Everest turbo. In: JR Sutton, G Coates and CS Houston (eds) *Hypoxia and Mountain Medicine*. Queen City Printers, Burlington, VT, pp. 202–12.

Shlim DR and Gallie J (1992) The causes of death among trekkers in Nepal. *Int J Sports Med.* **13(Suppl.)**: S74–6.

Ward MP, Milledge JS and West JB (2000) *High Altitude Medicine and Physiology* (3e). Arnold, London, pp. 22–32.

West JB (1993) Acclimatization and tolerance to extreme altitude. *J Wilderness Med.* **4**: 17–26.

2

High altitude illness

The term 'altitude illness' describes those medical conditions that are directly attributed to hypobaric hypoxia. Considerable overlap exists between these syndromes. However, it is convenient to separate them into three types, namely acute mountain sickness, high altitude cerebral oedema and high altitude pulmonary oedema (*see* Appendix 6, Fact sheet for altitude illness). Acute mountain sickness and high altitude cerebral oedema may represent different ends of the same disease process.

Acute mountain sickness (AMS)

Rapid ascent to altitudes above 2500 m often results in the syndrome known as acute mountain sickness (AMS). AMS is a collection of symptoms that appear gradually, typically 6–12 hours after arrival at high altitude, and usually resolve within one to three days if further ascent does not occur (*see* Appendix 3, Case histories). On occasion the onset of AMS may be delayed by 1–2 days following arrival at altitude.

The most important risk factors for the development of AMS are altitude gained (especially sleeping altitude) and rate of ascent. The prevalence of AMS among climbers in the Swiss Alps ranged from 9% at 2850 m to 53% at 4559 m (Maggiorini *et al.*, 1990). In the Mount Everest region of Nepal, approximately 50% of trekkers who walk to altitudes above 4000 m over five or more days develop AMS (Hackett *et al.*, 1976; Hackett and Rennie, 1979), while 84% of those who fly directly to 3860 m are affected (Murdoch, 1995a) (*see* Table 2.1). AMS is also being increasingly recognized at altitudes of between 1500 m and 2500 m. Males and females are affected similarly. There are few data on AMS in children, but current

Table 2.1: Incidence of AMS

(From various studies with different altitudes, rates of ascent and definitions of AMS)

Altitude (m)		Incidence (%)	Study
1900–2940	25	(Colorado)	Honigman et al., 1993
2000–2800	12	(Colorado)	Montgomery et al., 1989; Houston, 1985
2850	9	(Swiss Alps)	Maggiorini et al., 1990
3050	13	(Swiss Alps)	Maggiorini et al., 1990
3650	34	(Swiss Alps)	Maggiorini et al., 1990
4243	43–53	(Pheriche, Nepal)	Hackett and Rennie, 1979; Hackett et al., 1976
4394	67–77	(Mount Rainier, USA)	Larson et al., 1982; Ellsworth et al., 1987
4550	38.2	(Tuo-Tuo, Tibet)	Wu, 1994
4559	53	(Swiss Alps)	Maggiorini et al., 1990
4815	37	(Nepal)	Hirata et al., 1989
5400	63	(Thorong La, Nepal)	Kayser, 1991
5949	40	(Indian Himalaya)	Mistry et al., 1993
6195	30	(Mount McKinley [Denali], Alaska)	Hackett, 1980

information suggests that they are not at greater risk than adults. Exertion may be a risk factor for AMS, while lack of physical fitness is not. Some people have an inherent physiological susceptibility and readily develop AMS on high altitude exposure. These people should ascend at a slower rate, allowing more time for acclimatization.

There is no satisfactory test available that will predict who will get AMS, but one preliminary study has demonstrated that those with a hypersensitive gag reflex, extreme dizziness on hyperventilation or short breath-holding time are more susceptible (Austin and Sleigh, 1995). There is some evidence that measurements of cardiac and respiratory responses to hypoxia in a physiology laboratory may have some predictive value (Rathat et al., 1992; Savourey et al., 1995).

Symptoms and signs

The principal symptoms of AMS are headache, nausea, vomiting, anorexia, fatigue, dizziness and sleep disturbance, although all need not be present.

The characteristics of the headache are not sufficiently distinctive to differentiate it from other causes of headache. It is typically throbbing in nature, worse during the night and morning, aggravated by Valsalva's manoeuvre and stooping, may be either bitemporal or occipital, and can be very severe. Gastrointestinal disturbance is common, nausea and anorexia frequently being the predominant symptoms. Sleep disturbance is almost universal at high altitude, even without AMS, and is character- ized by difficulty initiating sleep, frequent wakening and periodic breathing (*see* page 36). However, these symptoms are often exaggerated during AMS. Profound apathy can result in the inability to perform basic tasks. The typical AMS sufferer has a headache, is off their food and has difficulty sleeping.

Box 2.1:   AMS symptoms

- Headache

- Nausea

- Vomiting

- Fatigue

- Anorexia

- Dizziness

- Sleep disturbance

There is a paucity of specific physical findings, especially in mild AMS. Blood pressure remains within the normal range, although it may be higher or lower than individual sea-level recordings. There is usually a mild tachycardia, and occasionally body temperature is raised (Maggiorini *et al.*, 1997). Crackles localized to one area of the chest are common and, especially in the presence of respiratory symptoms, should alert the ex- aminer to the possibility of high altitude pulmonary oedema (*see* page 17). Absence of the normal diuresis experienced at high altitude is charac- teristic. Peripheral oedema is common at high altitude (Hackett and Rennie, 1979), but may be more common among those with AMS.

The lack of specific symptoms and signs of AMS can result in diagnostic confusion with other conditions such as exhaustion, dehydration, hypothermia, alcoholic hangover, migraine and viral infections. In most cases, it is best to be conservative and, if there is any doubt, to treat the person as if they have AMS, but still keep an open mind about alternative diagnoses. Symptom scores have been developed which are mainly used for AMS research, but which may be helpful in the clinical setting (*see* Appendix 2).

Natural history

Symptoms of AMS usually resolve within one to three days if further ascent does not occur. Descent to low altitude effectively and rapidly reverses AMS. It should be remembered that AMS represents the mild end of the spectrum of acute altitude illness. The major concern is that it may progress to life-threatening high altitude cerebral and/or pulmonary oedema.

Mechanisms of AMS and HACE

The exact mechanism that causes AMS and HACE (high altitude cerebral oedema) is unknown, although the evidence points to a central nervous system process. It is possible that mild cerebral oedema is responsible for the symptoms of AMS, and that AMS and HACE represent different ends of the spectrum of a single disease process. A recent hypothesis is that hypoxaemia elicits various neurohumoral and haemodynamic responses that ultimately lead to elevated cerebral blood flow, altered blood–brain barrier permeability and cerebral oedema (*see* Figure 2.1). These changes result in brain swelling and raised intracranial pressure. According to this model, AMS occurs in individuals with inadequate cerebrospinal capacity to buffer the brain swelling. Those with a higher ratio of cranial cerebrospinal fluid (CSF) to brain volume are better able to compensate for swelling through CSF displacement, and are less likely to develop AMS.

Prevention

There are two principal methods of preventing or minimizing AMS:

1 graded ascent
2 drug prophylaxis.

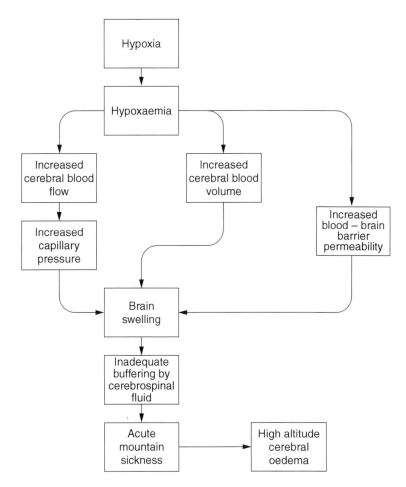

Figure 2.1: Pathogenesis of high altitude cerebral oedema. Reproduced with permission from Elsevier, *Lancet* (2003) **361**: 1967–74.

AMS is best prevented by slow, graded ascent, allowing time for acclimatization to occur. One current recommendation is that above 3000 m each night should average not more than 300 m above the last, with a rest day every two or three days (or every 1000 m). This formula emphasizes sleeping altitudes. This means that it is possible to ascend further than 300 m within a day so long as descent occurs prior to sleeping ('climb high, sleep low'). If a height difference between consecutive sleeping sites of more than 300 m is unavoidable, the ascent rate over subsequent days should be reduced so that the average daily ascent is 300 m. Thus if 600 m are climbed within one day, the next day should be a rest day involving no height gain. This recommendation was derived for trekkers in the Mount Everest region of Nepal, where it is well suited. For other areas of the world this schedule may appear painfully slow, and many people are clearly able to tolerate a more rapid ascent rate. Some authorities have recommended ascending no faster than 600 m per day (Hackett and Roach, 2001), and it is likely that a recommended ascent rate of no more than 400–600 m per day will be suitable for most people. The most important thing is to allow sufficient time, so that the ascent rate can be slowed if the need arises. Ascent should not occur while experiencing symptoms of AMS, and descent should be considered until symptoms are relieved, because of the risk that life-threatening complications may supervene.

In some situations, pharmacological prophylaxis of AMS is warranted. Opinions vary greatly as to who should and who should not receive drug prophylaxis, but the decision needs to be made on a case-by-case basis. It certainly should be considered when a large and rapid height gain is to be undertaken, as in an emergency, and for individuals with a history of increased susceptibility to altitude illness. Many choose to use regular drug prophylaxis against AMS, although it should be emphasized that careful planning to incorporate regular rest days and to avoid rapid ascents usually obviates the need for the use of drugs.

Acetazolamide

The carbonic anhydrase inhibitor, acetazolamide, is the drug of choice for prophylaxis (Birmingham Medical Research Expeditionary Society Mountain Sickness Study Group, 1981). By increasing renal bicarbonate excretion it produces a metabolic acidosis and stimulates respiration. It helps to maintain oxygenation during sleep and prevents periods of extreme hypoxaemia. Many dose regimens have been effective, the most common being 250 mg twice daily or 500 mg once daily of the slow-release preparation, starting at least 24 hours before ascent above 2500 m. Some have advocated doses as low as 125 mg twice daily, although pre-liminary clinical trial data are inconsistent. A recent meta-analysis concluded that daily prophylactic doses of less than 750 mg were ineffective (Dumont *et al.*, 2000). This claim runs contrary to clinical experience, and probably reflects the strict inclusion criteria in this review and the fact that studies with different ascent rates were compared. Prophylaxis should continue until either maximum ascent is reached or adequate acclimatization is judged to have occurred. Related drugs such as benzolamide (which does not cross the blood–brain barrier) prevent AMS and seem to have fewer side-effects, but are not yet available outside clinical trials.

Side-effects of acetazolamide are common and have been demonstrated to be unacceptable in a minority of individuals. Most notable are mild diuresis and paraesthesiae. Both tend to diminish with continued use. Paraesthesiae are most noticeable in the hands and feet, especially on pressure points. Carbonated drinks may taste flat. Acetazolamide is a sulpha drug and carries the usual precautions about hypersensitivity. The prolonged use of acetazolamide on expeditions and long treks at altitude has not been studied. There is no evidence to suggest that the prophylactic use of acetazolamide masks symptoms of AMS. Some individuals have reported symptoms of AMS on abrupt cessation of prophylaxis, and this should probably be avoided until descent.

Dexamethasone
Dexamethasone has also been used as prophylaxis for AMS, but it is not as effective as acetazolamide (Rabold, 1992). Its mechanism of action is unknown, but unlike acetazolamide, dexamethasone does not aid acclimatization. Concerns regarding side-effects limit the use of dexamethasone to the treatment of altitude illness and situations where prophylaxis is needed in individuals who are intolerant of or allergic to acetazolamide. The recommended prophylactic dose for adults is 4 mg every six to eight hours. The optimal time to commence dexamethasone has not been established,

---

Box 2.2: AMS prevention

1 **Gradual ascent**
   Over 3000 m: (i) ascend on average no more than
                          400–600 m/day

                    (ii) take a rest day every 1000 m or three days

2 **Drug prophylaxis**
   Acetazolamide 250 mg bd or 500 mg SR od from at least one day
   prior to ascent, po

---

although the first dose should probably be taken at least 24 hours prior to ascent to high altitude. Symptoms of AMS may appear if dexamethasone is discontinued prior to acclimatization. Short-term use of dexamethasone for treatment of AMS is relatively free of side-effects, although steroid psychosis may occur in this setting and could compromise rescue attempts.

Other drugs

Preliminary studies have indicated that *Ginkgo biloba* may be a useful prophylactic agent against AMS, but further studies are needed to characterize its role more fully. Nifedipine has a role in the treatment, and probably prophylaxis, of high altitude pulmonary oedema (HAPE), but does not appear to prevent AMS (Hohenhaus *et al.*, 1994).

Treatment

The principles of treatment of AMS are as follows.

1   Stop further ascent.

2   Descend if there is no improvement or if the condition worsens.

3   Descend immediately if there are symptoms or signs of cerebral or pulmonary oedema.

Mild AMS can be treated with rest to facilitate acclimatization. This may take from one to four days. Ascent to a higher sleeping altitude in the presence of symptoms of AMS is absolutely contraindicated. Because of the possible progression to life-threatening altitude illness (cerebral or pulmonary oedema), an individual with AMS should never be left alone. Simple analgesics such as aspirin and paracetamol (acetaminophen) may relieve headache, but are often ineffective. Other non-steroidal anti-inflammatory drugs, such as ibuprofen, may be useful (Broome *et al.*, 1994). Antiemetics can be used for nausea and vomiting. Acetazolamide, 250 mg every eight hours, is helpful in established AMS, relieving symptoms and improving arterial oxygenation (Grissom *et al.*, 1992). Dexamethasone relieves symptoms of AMS but does not improve objective physiological abnormalities. It can be a useful adjunct to descent and other treatments in severe AMS (Rabold, 1992). Supplementary oxygen and treatment in a portable hyperbaric chamber are also often effective in relieving symptoms in conjunction with drugs to facilitate descent.

It cannot be overemphasized that descent remains the most important and only definitive treatment for all forms of altitude illness. *If there is any doubt, descend!* If symptoms worsen despite an additional 24 hours' acclimatization, descent is indicated. Two indications for immediate descent include abnormal neurological features (especially altered consciousness and ataxia) and pulmonary oedema. Descent should be to an altitude lower than that where symptoms began. If this is not possible, descent of only a few hundred metres may be sufficient to bring about improvement.

Box 2.3: AMS treatment

Mild:	Rest (stop further ascent)
	Simple analgesia/antiemetics as required
Moderate/severe:	Descent
	Oxygen
	Acetazolamide, 250 mg tds, po
	Dexamethasone, 4 mg qds, oral or iv
	Hyperbaric chamber

High altitude cerebral oedema (HACE)

High altitude cerebral oedema (HACE) is a rare but life-threatening form of altitude illness. Individuals with HACE have usually had symptoms of AMS (*see* Appendix 3, Case histories). Indeed, AMS and HACE probably represent two ends of a spectrum, the distinction between them being inherently blurred. Although it is more likely to occur above 3500 m, HACE has been described at altitudes as low as 2500 m. The prevalence of HACE is difficult to estimate because of the difficulty in determining the at-risk group, but it is probably 1–2% of those ascending to 4500 m.

Symptoms and signs

People with HACE become confused, disorientated, irrational, unusually quiet or noisy, clumsy with their hands, unsteady on their feet and begin to hallucinate. Eventually they become lethargic and sleepy before slipping into a coma. Clinical examination may reveal papilloedema, ataxia, focal neurological signs including cranial nerve palsy and hemiparesis, seizures, confusion and reduced conscious level. Retinal haemorrhages are common. The progression from initial symptoms to coma may take as little as 12 hours. Ataxia is one of the first signs to appear and can be readily tested by heel–toe walking. This is an important clinical test. Anyone unwell at high altitude who is ataxic without another obvious cause should be regarded as suffering from HACE until proven otherwise. The first signs to appear are usually the last to disappear, and consequently a HACE victim may be ataxic for some time after successful treatment. Concomitant pulmonary oedema is common, and HACE may rapidly develop in those with high altitude pulmonary oedema (HAPE), possibly due to increased hypoxaemia. As the progression from AMS to HACE is usually gradual, it can be difficult to decide when HACE is present. If there is any doubt, assume HACE is present.

Box 2.4: HACE symptoms and signs

- Usually preceded by AMS

- Ataxia

- Behaviour change

- Hallucination

- Disorientation

- Confusion

- Decreased level of consciousness

- Coma

Treatment

Anyone suffering from symptoms of HACE should descend immediately or death is a likely consequence. Dexamethasone, 8 mg initially followed by 4 mg every six hours (administered parenterally or orally if this is impractical), and oxygen (if available) should be given. Portable hyperbaric chambers can be very effective in treating HACE, although the beneficial effects may be only temporary (*see* page 22). Treatment with these devices should always be followed by descent. Their use may improve the patient's condition such that they can descend unaided rather than requiring assistance. Occasionally, immediate descent may not be possible. In this situation, management of HACE involves regular administration of dexamethasone and oxygen, and prolonged hyperbaric treatment while arranging evacuation. Acetazolamide may also be considered in the treatment of HACE, but there is no evidence that it is useful.

Prevention of HACE is the same as for AMS.

Box 2.5: HACE treatment

- **Descent**

- Oxygen

- Dexamethasone, 8 mg and then 4 mg six-hourly, oral, iv or im

- Hyperbaric chamber

High altitude pulmonary oedema (HAPE)

High altitude pulmonary oedema (HAPE) usually occurs in the first two to four days after ascent to altitudes above 2500 m. As many as 10% of those ascending very rapidly to 4500 m will develop HAPE (Bärtsch *et al.*, 1990), although incidences of 1–2% are more likely with standard ascent rates (*see* Table 2.2). HAPE may also develop on reascent to significant altitude by a high altitude resident after a stay at low altitude (*see* Appendix 3,

Case histories). It also occurs frequently in climbers who have acclimatized to altitudes of around 5000 m and who then make rapid ascents to 7000 m or higher. In adults it may be more common in men than in women, and is often associated with exertion. Some individuals are particularly susceptible and have suffered repeated episodes. There may be an increased risk of HAPE in individuals who suffer from respiratory viral infections during or before ascent (Durmowicz *et al.*, 1997). People with chronically increased pulmonary blood flow and/or pressure, such as occurs with unilateral absence of the right pulmonary artery or primary pulmonary hypertension, are at increased risk of HAPE, even at moderate altitudes (Hackett *et al.*, 1980; Naeije *et al.*, 1996).

As yet there is no satisfactory test to predict who will develop HAPE, but current research on pulmonary vascular response to hypoxia (measured by Doppler echocardiography) seems promising. The incidence of HAPE ranges from 0.0001% at 2700 m to more than 2% above 4000 m (*see* Table 2.2).

Table 2.2: Incidence of HAPE

(Various studies at different altitudes with different ascent schedules and definitions of HAPE)

Altitude (m)	Incidence (%)	Study
3500	0.57 (Leh, Ladakh)	Menon, 1965
3750	0.6 (La Oroya, Peru)	Hultgren and Marticorena, 1978
4243	2.5 (Pheriche, Nepal)	Hackett *et al.*, 1976
4400	0.5 (Mount Rainier, USA)	Houston, 1976
4550	1.27 (Tuo-Tuo, Tibet)	Wu, 1994
4559	11 (Swiss Alps)	Bärtsch *et al.*, 1990
3965–4423	0.44 (Mount Kenya)	Houston (cited by Hultgren, 1997)
6195	1 (Mount McKinley [Denali], Alaska)	Hackett, 1980

Symptoms and signs

HAPE may be preceded by symptoms of AMS, but often occurs without AMS. The first symptoms of HAPE are usually dyspnoea on exertion and reduced exercise tolerance, greater than expected for the altitude.

Climbing uphill is particularly problematic, and recovery from exercise is prolonged. This progresses to breathlessness at rest, especially at night. Cough, which is dry and annoying at first, becomes bubbly and wet with sputum that may be bloodstained. However, it should be noted that dry cough at high altitude is common (*see* page 39) and in most cases is not due to early HAPE.

Physical findings may be subtle initially. Tachycardia and tachypnoea are present at rest as the illness progresses, and right ventricular heave, prominent pulmonary second heart sound and features of right heart failure may be present. Fever is often present, but the temperature rarely exceeds 38.3°C (Maggiorini *et al.*, 1997). Crackles usually appear first in the right mid-lung field, and their distribution reflects the severity of illness. At high altitude, up to one-third of people with AMS and over 10% of those without AMS exhibit crackles on auscultation of the chest, despite an absence of respiratory symptoms. Whether this represents subclinical HAPE is unclear, although there is indirect evidence that this is relatively common (Cremona *et al.*, 2002). Many features of HAPE can be readily confused with pulmonary infarction or pneumonia.

Atypical presentations of HAPE occur not infrequently. Occasionally HAPE may appear dramatically without obvious preceding symptoms of AMS.

Box 2.6:   HAPE symptoms and signs

- May be preceded by AMS

- Dyspnoea

- Reduced exercise tolerance

- Dry cough

- Bloodstained sputum

- Crackles on auscultation

Mechanisms of HAPE

HAPE is a non-cardiogenic pulmonary oedema characterized by exaggerated pulmonary hypertension leading to capillary leakage through over-perfusion and/or stress failure. The reason for the accentuated pulmonary hypertension is unclear, although it is likely to be due to several factors (*see* Figure 2.2).

Inflammation is probably not a primary event in the pathogenesis of HAPE, although it may occur as a secondary event that results from alveolar flooding. Blunting of the clearance of alveolar fluid by the alveolar epithelium may predispose individuals to pulmonary oedema, and there is some indirect evidence to support this view.

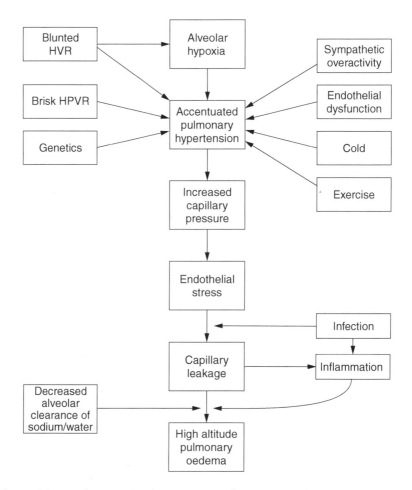

Figure 2.2:   Pathogenesis of HAPE. HVR = hypoxic ventilatory response; HPVR = hypoxic pulmonary vascular response. Reproduced with permission from Elsevier, *Lancet* (2003) **361**: 1967–74.

Treatment

Prognosis is directly related to severity of HAPE, and therefore early recognition is paramount. Death commonly results from incorrect diagnosis and failure to descend. Descent is the treatment of choice for anyone with HAPE, and should be initiated as soon as the condition is recognized. As with AMS, it is preferable to descend to below the altitude at which the patient was last free of symptoms of altitude illness. Exertion should be minimized, which may mean that the victim will need to be assisted and, if possible, they should be rescued in the upright or sitting position. Oxygen often produces immediate and dramatic improvement, and can be life-saving. Cold raises pulmonary artery pressure, and thus the patient should be kept warm.

Treatment in a portable hyperbaric chamber may relieve symptoms and facilitate descent, although the recumbent position necessary for operation may aggravate dyspnoea.

Several drugs have been used to treat HAPE, although their role should always be regarded as secondary, given the uniformly excellent response to descent and oxygen. Nifedipine, 10 mg sublingually (a capsule broken and held under the tongue), followed by 20 mg (slow-release preparation) by mouth four times daily, has been shown to help relieve symptoms and is the most useful (Oelz *et al.*, 1989). The sublingual dose may provoke systemic hypotension which may hamper descent and evacuation, and its use should probably be avoided. Other vasodilators, such as nitric oxide, hydralazine and phentolamine, are effective for HAPE but not practical for use in the field. Varying results have been obtained with frusemide, morphine and steroids such that none are currently recommended. Dexamethasone is usually given, as HAPE is often associated with HACE or AMS, and it may facilitate descent in this situation.

Individuals who have previously had an episode of HAPE must ascend cautiously on their next exposure to altitude, watching for the onset of symptoms. They should be prepared to descend if symptoms occur and carry nifedipine for treatment. The same measures for the prevention of AMS also apply to HAPE. In those with recurrent episodes of HAPE, one study supports the prophylactic use of nifedipine (20 mg slow release every eight hours) to prevent it (Bärtsch *et al.*, 1991), although it could be argued that those who are seriously susceptible to HAPE should not go high. The findings of a recent study indicated that inhaled β_2-agonists may be useful for the prevention of HAPE (Sartori *et al.*, 2002).

Box 2.7: HAPE treatment

- **Descent**
- Sit the patient upright
- Oxygen
- Nifedipine, 20 mg SR qds, po
- Hyperbaric chamber

The portable hyperbaric chamber

Portable hyperbaric chambers ('pressure bags') have become readily available over recent years, and their use has become a regular practice for the treatment of altitude illness. Constructed from lightweight fabric and inflated by foot- or hand-driven pumps, they provide rapid pressurization of patients to above ambient pressure, thus simulating descent. Continuous pumping is required to prevent the build-up of expired carbon dioxide, but the required pump rate may be reduced by the use of a lightweight carbon dioxide scrubber.

Three portable hyperbaric chambers are commercially available (*see* Figure 2.3). The Gamow bag is cylindrical in shape, measures 2.5 × 0.6 m and is inflated by a raft-style foot pump. Twelve pump strokes per minute are required to maintain the internal pressure of 104 mmHg and to prevent build-up of carbon dioxide. The total weight (including backpack and pump) is 6.5 kg. The CERTEC bag is conical, and measures 2.2 m in length and 0.65 m at its widest point. An internal pressure of 165 mmHg is maintained with a hand pump at a rate of 12 strokes per minute. At 4.8 kg (including mattress, pump, carry bag and tools for repair), it is lighter than the Gamow bag. The portable altitude chamber (PAC) has a tapered shape, is similar in size, weight and operating pressure to the Gamow bag, and is also operated by a foot pump. The PAC has easier access than other chambers, through a radial zipper at the head end, and is cheaper. All bags are acoustically transparent and have windows to allow visual contact with the patient. The companies that manufacture these bags

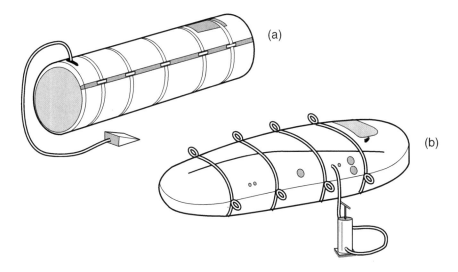

Figure 2.3:   Two portable hyperbaric chambers: (a) the Gamow bag; (b) the CERTEC bag.

have also produced larger multi-person portable hyperbaric chambers. The magnitude of simulated descent in a portable hyperbaric chamber depends on the type of chamber used and the actual altitude at which the treatment is taking place (*see* Figure 2.4).

Dramatic responses to hyperbaric treatment of AMS, HACE and HAPE have been reported. Controlled studies have shown that portable hyperbaric chambers relieve symptoms of AMS and improve arterial oxygenation (Bärtsch *et al.*, 1993; Keller *et al.*, 1995). A recent study concluded that some of the beneficial effects of the portable hyperbaric chamber are due to build-up of carbon dioxide (Imray *et al.*, 2001). Unfortunately, the beneficial effects usually disappear within 10 hours. Furthermore, patients with HAPE frequently do not tolerate the recumbent position necessary for operation. Raising the head end of the chamber by any means available may solve this problem. Given the relatively short-lived benefits, portable hyperbaric chambers should only be used when descent is not immediately possible, or to facilitate descent. There are no controlled data available to support any particular treatment schedule. However, pressurization for one to two hours is usually sufficient to facilitate descent and, if necessary, this can be repeated five to ten hours later.

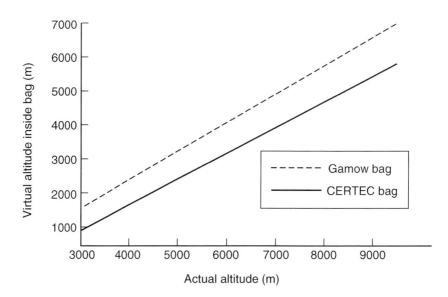

Figure 2.4: Graph showing simulated descent (virtual altitude) inside two types of hyperbaric bag which can be achieved at altitudes above 3000 m. (Reproduced with permission from Dubois C, Herry JP and Kayser B (1994) Portable hyperbaric medicine, some history. *J Wilderness Med.* **5**: 196. Published by Chapman & Hall.)

It is possible to hire rather than buy portable hyperbaric chambers in some parts of the world (e.g. Nepal). Sources for ordering portable hyperbaric chambers are listed at the end of this chapter (*see* page 33).

Subacute mountain sickness

Adults resident at low altitude who spend prolonged periods (months) at very high altitude (> 5500m) may develop signs and symptoms of congestive heart failure. This condition has been referred to as subacute mountain sickness, and its clinical features include oedema, dyspnoea, cough and exercise-induced angina. This illness is characterized by right ventricular hypertrophy, pericardial effusion, pulmonary hypertension (especially with exercise) and resolution of symptoms and signs with descent. Recommended treatment is descent with diuretics as adjunctive therapy (Anand *et al.*, 1990, 1993).

Chronic mountain sickness (Monge's disease)

Chronic mountain sickness (CMS) is a disorder of long-term high altitude residents, and is characterized by red cell counts higher than normally expected at high altitude, and hypoxaemia (Reeves and Weil, 2001). Originally described in South America, it has also been documented in high altitude residents in Colorado and in Han Chinese populations in Tibet.

Signs and symptoms reflect profound polycythaemia and hypoxaemia. Neuropsychological symptoms predominate, with headache, poor concentration, somnolence, dizziness and poor exercise tolerance. The high haemoglobin concentration and cyanosis combine to produce very dark lips and red, congested mucosal surfaces. Finger clubbing is often present.

Symptoms and signs disappear on descent to sea level. Venesection is useful.

Travelling with organized groups

Many tourists now trek to high altitude areas in organized groups with pre-arranged itineraries. This can be an excellent way to travel, especially for inexperienced walkers and for those seeking companionship. However, in Nepal concern has been raised about an association between trekking in this fashion and the development of altitude illness. While trekkers with organized groups have a similar incidence of AMS to individual trekkers (Murdoch, 1995a), their risk of dying from altitude illness is significantly greater (Shlim and Gallie, 1992). There are a number of possible reasons for this observation. Trekkers with organized groups have to keep pace with the rest of their group, and are often reluctant to admit to symptoms of AMS for fear of upsetting the plans of others or being left behind. This is compounded by peer pressure and tight itineraries that allow few deviations or additional rest days. Group leaders may be reluctant to diagnose altitude illness to avoid the logistic difficulties arising from an altered itinerary. These problems can be easily avoided. Itineraries should be designed such that ascent is gradual, and should include additional unscheduled days to allow alterations to the original plan if required. Trekking groups should be small, and members should be encouraged to mention symptoms when they appear. Group leaders should be able to recognize the symptoms and signs of altitude illness, and should keep a regular check on all members. Sick trekkers should always be in the company of a senior member of their trekking group. It is surprising how frequently people with significant altitude illness have been left on their own or in the care of local trekking staff.

Especially in high altitude areas of developing countries, trekking groups and mountaineering expeditions are often accompanied by local guides, porters, cooks and other staff. These people are also vulnerable to altitude illness and should be cared for in the same manner as group members.

By advising patients to choose a trek from a brochure which allows adequate time for acclimatization and rest days to allow for itinerary changes due to illness, doctors may prevent altitude sickness and swing the consumer demand in favour of safe trekking.

Box 2.8: Package-holiday treks

Choose treks that allow for:

- a safe ascent schedule

- planned rest days

Rapid motorized transport to high altitude

Road and air links allow the rapid transport of unacclimatized travellers to many high altitude areas of the world. This is most apparent in the Tibetan plateau and in the South American Andes, where it is possible to reach heights of over 5000 m within a few hours. The risk of altitude illness following such rapid ascent is high and, in some cases (especially Tibet), rapid descent to low altitude may be difficult if problems arise. Eighty per cent of workers at the astronomical observatory on Mauna Kea, Hawaii (4205 m) suffered from AMS after driving up from sea level (Forster, 1985). Of tourists flying directly to Hotel Everest View in Nepal

(3860 m), 84% developed AMS (Murdoch, 1995b). Obviously, the best preventative measure is to avoid such rapid ascent. For those who choose to undertake this type of travel, acetazolamide prophylaxis should be considered and exertion should be minimized during the first few days after arrival at altitude.

Box 2.9: Rapid ascent by road or air

- Avoid if possible
- Minimize exertion during the first few days after arrival at high altitude

---

References and further reading

Acute mountain sickness

Austin D and Sleigh J (1995) Prediction of acute mountain sickness. *BMJ*. **311**: 989–90.

Barry PW and Pollard AJ (2003) Altitude illness. *BMJ*. **326**: 915–19.

Basnyat B and Murdoch DR (2003) High-altitude illness. *Lancet*. **361**: 1967–74.

Birmingham Medical Research Expeditionary Society Mountain Sickness Study Group (1981) Acetazolamide in control of acute mountain sickness. *Lancet*. **i**: 180–3.

Broome JR, Stoneham MD, Beeley JM *et al*. (1994) High altitude headache: treatment with ibuprofen. *Aviat Space Environ Med*. **65**: 19–20.

Collier DJ, Rosenberg ME, Cifuentes L *et al*. (1998) Actions of carbonic anhydrase inhibitors in man. *Br J Clin Pharmacol*. **491**: 200.

Dickinson J, Heath D, Gosney J *et al*. (1983) Altitude-related deaths in seven trekkers in the Himalayas. *Thorax*. **38**: 646–56.

Dumont L, Mardirosoff C and Tramèr MR (2000) Efficacy and harm of pharmacological prevention of acute mountain sickness: quantitative systematic review. *BMJ*. **321**: 267–72.

Ellsworth AJ, Larson EB and Strickland D (1987) A randomized trial of dexamethasone and acetazolamide for acute mountain sickness prophylaxis. *Am J Med*. **83**: 1024–30.

Grissom CK, Roach RC, Sarnquist FH *et al*. (1992) Acetazolamide in the treatment of acute mountain sickness: clinical efficacy and effect on gas exchange. *Ann Intern Med*. **116**: 461–5.

Hackett PH (1980) *Mountain Sickness: prevention, recognition and treatment*. American Alpine Club, New York.

Hackett PH (1999) The cerebral etiology of high-altitude cerebral edema and acute mountain sickness. *Wild Environ Med*. **10**: 97–109.

Hackett PH and Rennie D (1979) Rales, peripheral edema, retinal hemorrhage and acute mountain sickness. *Am J Med*. **67**: 214–18.

Hackett PH and Roach RC (2001) High-altitude illness. *NEJM*. **345**: 107–14.

Hackett PH, Rennie D and Levine HD (1976) The incidence, importance, and prophylaxis of acute mountain sickness. *Lancet*. **ii**: 1149–54.

Hirata K, Masuyama S and Saito A (1989) Obesity as a risk factor for acute mountain sickness. *Lancet*. **28**: 1040–1.

Hohenhaus E, Niroomand F, Georre S *et al*. (1994) Nifedipine does not prevent acute mountain sickness. *Am J Resp Crit Care Med*. **150**: 857–60.

Honigman B, Thesis MK and Koziol-McLain J (1993) Acute mountain sickness in a general tourist population at moderate altitude. *Ann Intern Med*. **118**: 587–92.

Houston CS (1985) Incidence of acute mountain sickness: a study of winter visitors to six Colorado ski resorts. *Am Alpine J*. **27**: 162–5.

Johnson TS and Rock PB (1988) Acute mountain sickness. *NEJM*. **319**: 841–5.

Kayser B (1991) Acute mountain sickness in western tourists around the Thorong pass (5400 m) in Nepal. *J Wilderness Med*. **2**: 110–17.

Larson EB, Roach RC, Schoene RB *et al*. (1982) Acute mountain sickness and acetazolamide – clinical efficacy and effect on ventilation. *JAMA*. **248**: 328–32.

Maggiorini M, Bühler B, Walter M *et al.* (1990) Prevalence of acute mountain sickness in the Swiss Alps. *BMJ.* **301**: 853–5.

Maggiorini M, Bärtsch P and Oelz O (1997) Association between raised body temperature and acute mountain sickness: cross-sectional study. *BMJ.* **315**: 403–4.

Milledge JS (1983) Acute mountain sickness. *Thorax.* **38**: 641–5.

Mistry G, Chandrashekhar Y, Sen U *et al.* (1993) Study of acute mountain sickness during rapid ascent. *J Assoc Physicians India.* **41**: 500–2.

Montgomery AB, Mills J and Luce JM (1989) Incidence of acute mountain sickness at intermediate altitude. *JAMA.* **261**: 732–4.

Pollard AJ (1992) Altitude-induced illness. *BMJ.* **304**: 1324–5.

Rabold MB (1992) Dexamethasone for prophylaxis and treatment of acute mountain sickness. *J Wilderness Med.* **3**: 54–60.

Rathat C, Richalet JP, Herry JP *et al.* (1992) Detection of high-risk subjects for high-altitude diseases. *Int J Sports Med.* **13**: 76–8.

Roach RC and Hackett PH (2001) Frontiers of hypoxia research: acute mountain sickness. *J Exp Biol.* **204**: 3161–70.

Roach RC, Bärtsch P, Hackett PH *et al.* (1993) The Lake Louise acute mountain sickness scoring system. In: JR Sutton, CS Houston and G Coates (eds) *Hypoxia and Molecular Medicine.* Queen City Printers, Burlington, VT.

Savourey G, Moirant C, Eterradossi J *et al.* (1995) Acute mountain sickness relates sea-level partial pressure of oxygen. *Eur J Appl Physiol.* **70**: 469–76.

Singh I, Khanna PK, Srivastava MC *et al.* (1969) Acute mountain sickness. *NEJM.* **280**: 175–84.

Wu T (1994) Children on the Tibetan Plateau. *Newsletter Int Soc Mountain Med.* **4**: 5–7.

Wu TY (1987) An epidemiological study on high altitude disease at Qinghai-Xizang (Tibet) plateau. *Chin J Epidemiol.* **8**: 65–9.

HACE

Hackett PH (1999) The cerebral etiology of high-altitude cerebral edema and acute mountain sickness. *Wild Environ Med*. **10**: 97–109.

Hackett PH and Roach RC (2001) High-altitude illness. *NEJM*. **345**: 107–14.

Houston CS and Dickinson J (1975) Cerebral form of high-altitude illness. *Lancet*. **ii**: 758–61.

Ravenhill TH (1913) Some experiences of mountain sickness in the Andes. *J Trop Med Hygiene*. **16**: 314–20.

HAPE

Bärtsch P, Vock P, Maggiorini M *et al*. (1990) Respiratory symptoms radiographic and physiologic correlations at high altitude. In: JR Sutton, G Coates and JE Remmers (eds) *Hypoxia: the adaptations*. DC Decker Inc, Burlington, Ontario, Canada.

Bärtsch P, Maggiorini M, Ritter M *et al*. (1991) Prevention of high-altitude pulmonary edema by nifedipine. *NEJM*. **325**: 1284–9.

Cremona G, Asnaghi R, Baderna P *et al*. (2002) Pulmonary extravascular fluid accumulation in recreational climbers: a prospective study. *Lancet*. **359**: 303–9.

Durmowicz AG, Noordeweir E, Nicholas R *et al*. (1997) Inflammatory processes may predispose children to high-altitude pulmonary edema. *J Pediatr*. **130**: 838–40.

Hackett PH and Roach RC (1990) High altitude pulmonary edema. *J Wilderness Med*. **1**: 3–26.

Hackett PH and Roach RC (2001) High-altitude illness. *NEJM*. **345**: 107–14.

Hackett PH, Creagh CE, Grover RF *et al*. (1980) High-altitude pulmonary edema in persons without the right pulmonary artery. *NEJM*. **302**: 1070–3.

Houston C (1976) High altitude illness: disease with protean manifestations. *JAMA*. **236**: 21–93.

Houston CS (1960) Acute pulmonary edema of high altitude. *NEJM*. **263**: 478–80.

Hultgren H (1997) High altitude pulmonary edema. In: H Hultgren (ed.) *High Altitude Medicine*. Hultgren Publications, Stanford, CA.

Hultgren HN and Marticorena EA (1978) High altitude pulmonary edema: epidemiologic observations in Peru. *Chest.* **74**: 372–6.

Jerome EH and Severinghaus JW (1996) High altitude pulmonary edema. *NEJM.* **334**: 662–3.

Menon ND (1965) High altitude pulmonary edema: a clinical study. *NEJM.* **273**: 66–73.

Naeije R, De Backer D, Vachiéry J-L *et al.* (1996) High-altitude pulmonary edema with primary pulmonary hypertension. *Chest.* **110**: 286–9.

Oelz O, Maggiorini M, Ritter M *et al.* (1989) Nifedipine for high altitude pulmonary oedema. *Lancet.* **ii**: 1241–4.

Peacock AJ (1995) High altitude pulmonary oedema: who gets it and why? *Eur Respir J.* **8**: 1819–21.

Richalet JP (1995) High altitude pulmonary oedema: still a place for controversy? *Thorax.* **50**: 923–9.

Sartori C, Allemann Y, Duplain H *et al.* (2002) Salmeterol for the prevention of high-altitude pulmonary edema. *NEJM.* **346**: 1631–6.

Swenson ER, Maggiorini M, Mongovin S *et al.* (2002) Pathogenesis of high-altitude pulmonary edema. Inflammation is not an etiologic factor. *JAMA.* **287**: 2228–35.

West JB, Colice GL, Lee YJ *et al.* (1995) Pathogenesis of high-altitude pulmonary oedema: direct evidence of stress failure of pulmonary capillaries. *Eur Respir J.* **8**: 523–9.

Portable hyperbaric chamber

Bärtsch P, Merki B, Hofstetter D *et al.* (1993) Treatment of acute mountain sickness by simulated descent: a randomised controlled trial. *BMJ.* **306**: 1098–101.

Dubois C, Herry JP and Kayser B (1994) Portable hyperbaric medicine, some history. *J Wilderness Med.* **5**: 190–8.

Imray CHE, Clarke T, Forster PJG *et al.* (2001) Carbon dioxide contributes to the beneficial effect of pressurization in a portable hyperbaric chamber at high altitude. *Clin Sci.* **100**: 151–7.

Keller HR, Maggiorini M, Bärtsch P *et al.* (1995) Simulated descent *v* dexamethasone in treatment of acute mountain sickness: a randomised trial. *BMJ.* **310**: 1232–5.

Subacute mountain sickness

Anand IS, Malhotra RM, Chandrashekar Y *et al.* (1990) Adult subacute mountain sickness: a syndrome of congestive heart failure in man at very high altitude. *Lancet.* **335**: 561–5.

Anand IS, Chandrashekar Y, Rao SK *et al.* (1993) Body fluid compartments, renal blood flow and hormones at 6000 m in normal subjects. *J Appl Physiol.* **74**: 1234–9.

Chronic mountain sickness

Heath D and Williams DR (1995) Monge's disease. In: *High Altitude Medicine and Pathology* (4e). Oxford University Press, Oxford.

Monge CC and Whittembury J (1976) Chronic mountain sickness. *Johns Hopkins Med J.* **139**: 87–9.

Pei SX, Chen XJ, Si Ren BZ *et al.* (1989) Chronic mountain sickness in Tibet. *Q J Med.* **71**: 555–74.

Reeves JT and Weil JV (2001) Chronic mountain sickness. A view from the crow's nest. *Adv Exp Med Biol.* **502**: 419–37.

Travelling with organized groups

Murdoch DR (1995a) Symptoms of infection and altitude illness among hikers in the Mount Everest region of Nepal. *Aviat Space Environ Med.* **66**: 148–51.

Shlim DR and Gallie J (1992) The causes of death among trekkers in Nepal. *Int J Sports Med.* **13(Suppl.)**: S74–6.

Rapid transport to high altitude

Forster PJ (1985) Effect of different ascent profiles on performance at 4200 m elevation. *Aviat Space Environ Med.* **56**: 758–64.

Murdoch DR (1995b) Altitude illness among tourists flying to 3740 meters elevation in the Nepal Himalayas. *J Travel Med.* **2**: 255–6.

Portable hyperbaric chambers – sales and rental

France

Le Caisson Hyperbare (sales and rental)
CERTEC
Sourcieux-les-Mines
69210 L'Arbresle
France
Tel: 00 33 4 74 70 39 82
Fax: 00 33 4 74 70 37 66
Website: www.certec.fr

USA

The Gamow Bag
Chinook Medical Gear, Inc.
120 Rock Point Drive
Unit C
Durango
CO 81301
USA
Tel: 001 970 375 1241
Fax: 001 970 375 6343
Website: www.chinookmed.com

Australia
The PAC (Portable Altitude Chamber)
Himalayan Medical Supplies
PO Box 53
Repton
NSW 2454
Australia
Tel: (02) 6653 4241
Fax: (02) 6655 0266
Email: pac@treksafe.com.au
Website: www.treksafe.com.au

3

Other altitude related disorders

Peripheral oedema

Peripheral oedema, especially involving the hands and face, is common at high altitude (18% in one report), and is twice as common in women (Hackett and Rennie, 1979). The incidence is slightly higher among those with AMS. Treatment is not usually necessary, but diuretics (in the absence of symptoms of AMS) have been used.

High altitude retinal haemorrhage

Disc hyperaemia, vascular engorgement and tortuosity, and retinal haemorrhage are the retinal changes associated with ascent to high altitude. Retinal haemorrhages occur in 30–35% of trekkers at 5000 m. They are less common in those with previous high altitude exposure and in high altitude natives. Possible risk factors for the development of these haemorrhages are rapid ascent, Valsalva's manoeuvre (coughing and straining), polycythaemia and raised intra-ocular pressure. The haemorrhages may occur in the deep layer of the retina, in which case they are round in shape. More superficial haemorrhages are flame-shaped.

Retinal haemorrhages are usually asymptomatic and are likely to resolve rapidly and spontaneously. Field defects are rarely reported. However, some individuals have developed scotomata that have not resolved. Individuals with haemorrhages involving the macula area are particularly likely to develop visual deficit. Although descent might be advisable, no specific treatment is available.

Sleep and periodic breathing

Sleep is of poor quality at altitude, with a decrease in quantity of both deep sleep and rapid eye movement (REM) sleep. Periodic breathing, characterized by repeated episodes of hyperpnoea followed by apnoea, is a common occurrence at high altitude. Awareness of periodic breathing varies considerably, ranging from complete unawareness to repeated wakening in a panicked state following an apnoeic episode. Many people have woken thinking they are being suffocated. Oxygen desaturations accompany periodic breathing (Salvaggio *et al.*, 1998).

Periodic breathing is not clearly related to altitude illness (Eichenberger *et al.*, 1996), and tends to lessen with time at high altitude. There is some evidence to suggest that people with high hypoxic ventilatory responses (who tend to acclimatize faster and suffer less from altitude illness) have more periodic breathing, while those with low hypoxic ventilatory responses have more even breathing and will suffer fewer periods of extreme hypoxaemia. Acetazolamide is a very effective treatment, and can be given as a single night-time dose of 250 mg by mouth. It reduces the amount of periodic breathing and improves arterial oxygen saturation in sleep (Hackett and Rennie, 1976).

There are conflicting reports about the effects of benzodiazepines on sleep and oxygen saturation, but the decrease in oxygen saturations observed in some studies suggests that these drugs should not be recommended for routine use at altitude (Dubowitz, 1998; Roggla *et al.*, 2000).

Neurological disorders at high altitude

In addition to HACE, a number of neurological conditions have been described at high altitude in the absence of concomitant altitude illness. Several mountaineers have developed focal neurological events while at high altitude, typically at heights above 5500 m. Most have taken the form of transient ischaemic attacks involving the middle cerebral artery territory and have resolved with descent, but permanent loss of function has been documented. It is unknown whether these events have a haemorrhagic, thrombotic or vasospastic pathogenesis, but it is possible that all three occur. Severe hyperviscosity has been measured among climbers to extreme altitude, and may also play a role.

Other types of focal neurological deficits have also been reported, including cranial nerve palsies, cortical blindness, hemianopia, amaurosis fugax, unilateral paraesthesiae and dysphasia. Again the pathogenesis is uncertain, and most have been transient in nature.

Regardless of cause, immediate descent and administration of oxygen (if available) are recommended. In addition, dexamethasone should be used as for HACE. Although the use of aspirin as an anti-platelet agent might be considered logical (and has been used), the common finding of retinal haemorrhage at altitude and the cerebral haemorrhages seen at post-mortem in specimens from HACE victims may persuade otherwise. However, there is currently no evidence that the use of aspirin has adverse effects in these situations. Carbon dioxide breathing has afforded prompt relief for cortical blindness (Hackett *et al.*, 1987), and may be useful for other focal neurological conditions, but its use remains controversial.

The natural history of migraine at high altitude is incompletely understood. In South America, a higher prevalence of migraine in high altitude populations has been documented (Arregui *et al.*, 1991). Anecdotal reports suggest that migrainous attacks have been triggered by exposure to hypobaric hypoxia. Moreover, severe focal neurological symptoms, including hemiparesis and dysphasia, have been associated with migraine attacks at high altitude in people who have not experienced these symptoms during attacks at sea level (Jenzer and Bärtsch, 1993; Murdoch, 1995a). It is possible that many transient focal neurological deficits occurring at high altitude may have a migrainous aetiology. Until more information is available, descent is again recommended for any significant neurological symptoms developing at high altitude.

Exposure to extreme altitude may cause transient neurological deficits affecting motor, sensory and higher functions such as memory and cognition. These effects may contribute to injury and death which would normally be avoided by experienced mountaineers at lower altitudes. Residual neurological deficits (motor co-ordination and memory) persisting for at least one year following extreme altitude exposure have been documented.

Thrombosis

Cerebral and peripheral venous thrombosis and cases of pulmonary embolism have been reported at high altitude, especially above 6000 m (Ward, 1975). Risk factors include cold, dehydration and decreased physical activity (e.g. while tent bound in bad weather). Raised haematocrit and increased blood viscosity may also contribute. There do not appear to be changes in the coagulation cascade or in platelet count or function due to hypoxia, although changes suggestive of disseminated intravascular coagulation have been noted in patients with altitude illness.

Prevention is clearly important. The body (especially limbs) should be protected from cold, and regular limb movement during periods of inactivity should be performed. Adequate hydration should be maintained, and oxygen may benefit those with cerebral thrombosis or pulmonary embolism. Anyone experiencing a thrombotic episode at altitude should descend.

High altitude anxiety

Many people become anxious on ascent to high altitude, frightened that they will develop life-threatening altitude illness. This is more common during first high altitude exposures and following a previous unpleasant experience at high altitude. Many trek leaders have noted an increasing prevalence of this condition among their clients over the years, coinciding with the greater availability of information about high altitude medical problems. Typical clinical features include shortness of breath, dizziness and hyperventilation. Arterial oxygen saturation is normal for the altitude, there are typically no abnormalities on chest auscultation and there may be a surprisingly rapid response to oxygen or hyperbaric treatment. Although in certain circumstances anxiety may be considered, it is difficult to exclude altitude illness with confidence. Consequently, in such cases it is safer to assume altitude illness as the working diagnosis until proven otherwise. One study suggested that anxiety was a predictor for the development of AMS (Missoum et al., 1992).

High altitude cough

Most cases of cough and sore throat at altitude do not have an obvious infectious aetiology. An increase in cough frequency and an increased sensitivity of cough receptors (following acclimatization) have been documented at altitude (Barry *et al.*, 1997). Increased ventilation, dry cold air and mouth-breathing dry the respiratory mucosa, presumably leading to high altitude cough. Resetting of central cough receptors has also been suggested as a mechanism.

Cough can be disabling and has been severe enough to cause rib fractures. Breathing through a silk scarf or balaclava may alleviate symptoms, as may the use of a humidification mask similar to the heat and moisture exchanger or 'artificial nose' used in anaesthesia. However, all of these methods have been associated with the sensation of dyspnoea or suffocation, possibly by increasing the work of breathing. Many climbers gain relief from high altitude sore throat by using throat lozenges. Cold-induced rhinorrhoea is also common among high altitude travellers (Silvers, 1991).

Infections at high altitude

Travellers have long noted that infections are common at high altitudes and are often slow to resolve. Among high altitude trekkers in Nepal, 87% experience at least one symptom suggestive of infection: 75% develop coryza, 42% develop cough, 39% develop sore throat and 36% develop diarrhoea (Murdoch, 1995b). These symptoms are more common among those with AMS, and there is further evidence to suggest that inflammatory processes (e.g. viral respiratory tract infection) may predispose children to high altitude pulmonary oedema (Durmowicz *et al.*, 1997). Frequently, descent has proved to be a necessary adjunct to other treatment options. The effect of a high altitude environment on the immune response has not been studied extensively, but the information available suggests that susceptibility to bacterial infections is increased while the response to viruses is unchanged (Meehan, 1987). People with infections should consider ascending at a slower rate. If the infection is severe, descent is recommended until the symptoms have improved.

High altitude deterioration and appetite

The term 'high altitude deterioration' refers to a general deterioration in physical condition and lack of further acclimatization occurring after lengthy stays at extreme altitude. Although there is considerable individual variation, it usually occurs at altitudes above 5500 m. Typical features include progressive weight loss, worsening appetite, poor sleep and increasing lethargy. Although the underlying mechanism is unknown, it can be brought about by hypobaric hypoxia *per se*, and can be aggravated by other factors such as dehydration and starvation. Exposure to altitudes above 5000 m appears to be associated with decreased appetite, even in individuals who are otherwise well (Westerterp-Plantenga *et al.*, 1999; Westerterp, 2001).

References and further reading

Arregui A, Cabrera J, Leon-Velarde F *et al.* (1991) High prevalence of migraine in a high-altitude population. *Neurology.* **41**: 1668–70.

Barry PW, Mason NP, Riordan M *et al.* (1997) Cough frequency and cough-receptor sensitivity are increased in man at altitude. *Clin Sci.* **93**: 181–6.

Basnyat B, Cumbo TA and Edelman R (2000) Acute medical problems in the Himalayas outside the setting of altitude sickness. *High Alt Med Biol.* **1**: 167–74.

Bonnon M, Noël-Jorand M-C and Therme P (1995) Psychological changes during altitude hypoxia. *Aviat Space Environ Med.* **66**: 330–5.

Dubowitz G (1998) Effect of temazepam on oxygen saturation and sleep quality at high altitude: randomised placebo controlled crossover trial. *BMJ.* **316**: 587–9.

Durmowicz AG, Noordeweir E, Nicholas R *et al.* (1997) Inflammatory processes may predispose children to high-altitude pulmonary edema. *J Pediatr.* **130**: 838–40.

Eichenberger U, Weiss E, Riemann D *et al*. (1996) Nocturnal periodic breathing and the development of acute high altitude illnesses. *Am J Respir Crit Care Med*. **154**: 1748–54.

Hackett PH and Rennie D (1976) The incidence, importance and prophylaxis of acute mountain sickness. *Lancet*. **2**: 1149–55.

Hackett PH and Rennie D (1979) Rales, peripheral edema, retinal hemorrhage and acute mountain sickness. *Am J Med*. **67**: 214–18.

Hackett PH, Hollingsmead KF, Roach R *et al*. (1987) Cortical blindness in high altitude climbers and trekkers: a report of six cases. In: J Sutton, C Houston and G Coates (eds) *Hypoxia and Cold*. Praeger Press, New York.

Hornbein TF, Townes BD, Schoene RB *et al*. (1989) The cost to the central nervous system of climbing to extremely high altitude. *NEJM*. **321**: 1714–19.

Jenzer G and Bärtsch P (1993) Migraine with aura at high altitude. *J Wilderness Med*. **4**: 412–15.

Meehan RT (1987) Immune suppression at high altitude. *Ann Emerg Med*. **16**: 974–9.

Missoum G, Rosnet E and Richalet J-P (1992) Control of anxiety and acute mountain sickness in Himalayan mountaineers. *Int J Sports Med*. **13(Suppl. 1)**: 537–9.

Murdoch DR (1995a) Focal neurological deficits and migraine at high altitude. *J Neurol Neurosurg Psychiatry*. **58**: 637.

Murdoch DR (1995b) Symptoms of infection and altitude illness among hikers in the Mount Everest region of Nepal. *Aviat Space Environ Med*. **66**: 148–51.

Regard M, Oelz O, Brugger P *et al*. (1989) Persistent cognitive impairment in climbers after repeated exposure to extreme altitude. *Neurology*. **39**: 210–13.

Roggla G, Moser B and Roggla M (2000) Effect of temazepam on ventilatory response at moderate altitude. *BMJ*. **320**: 56.

Salvaggio A, Insalaco G, Marrone O *et al*. (1998) Effects of high-altitude periodic breathing on sleep and arterial oxyhaemoglobin saturation. *Eur Respir J*. **12**: 408–13.

Silvers WS (1991) The skier's nose: a model of cold-induced rhinorrhea. *Ann Allergy*. **67**: 32–6.

Sutton JR (1983) High altitude retinal hemorrhage. *Semin Respir Med.* **5**: 159–63.

Ward M (1954) High altitude deterioration. *Proc R Soc Lond.* **143**: 40–2.

Ward M (1975) *Mountain Medicine.* Crosby, Lockwood and Staples, London.

Weil JV (1985) Sleep at high altitude. *Clin Chest Med.* **6**: 615–21.

Westerterp KR (2001) Energy and water balance at high altitude. *News Physiol Sci.* **16**: 134–7.

Westerterp-Plantenga MS, Westerterp KR, Rubbens M *et al.* (1999) Appetite at 'high altitude' [Operation Everest III (Comex-'97)]: a simulated ascent of Mount Everest. *J Appl Physiol.* **87**: 391–9.

Wohns RN (1986) Transient ischaemic attacks at high altitude. *Crit Care Med.* **14**: 517–18.

4

Children at altitude

Children increasingly visit high altitudes as the popularity of family treks rises and school expeditions take the young to remote high regions. A much larger number of low altitude children travel to moderate altitude at resorts in Europe and especially North America. Other children accompany their parents who work in various high altitude regions, notably in the South American ranges. There is very little population-based information about the problems that affect children at high altitude, and although serious altitude disorders are uncommon, AMS, HAPE and HACE may all occur in the young. The study of altitude illness in children is further complicated by the fact that the non-specific symptoms of altitude illness are particularly difficult to recognize in early childhood. These issues have been considered in detail by an international ad hoc Committee on Children at Altitude organized by the International Society for Mountain Medicine (Pollard *et al.*, 2001).

AMS in children

In the past, anecdotal reports have suggested that AMS is more common in children, but there is little evidence to support this observation. The majority of carefully conducted studies reported in the past decade suggest that AMS in children is no more common than AMS in adults (*see* Table 4.1). However, some controversy still exists, and one small study found much higher rates of AMS in both teenagers and young children than in adults (Moraga *et al.*, 2002). The significance of this finding is unclear since, as in most other studies, there was no low altitude control group. However, it could suggest that rates of altitude illness in children are affected differently from those in adults in some populations or following certain ascent schedules. A modified AMS score (the Children's Lake Louise score (CLLS); *see* Appendix 2) has been developed and validated for use in preverbal children (under 3 years of age), and further studies using this scoring system may help to clarify this issue (Yaron *et al.*, 1997). The CLLS has a high level of inter-observer agreement when used by parents, and it may be helpful in educating parents about the symptoms of AMS (Yaron *et al.*, 2002).

Table 4.1: Reports of incidence of AMS and HAPE in children (adapted with permission from Pollard *et al.*, 2001)

Location, altitude	Number of children (age)	Number of adults	AMS in children	AMS in adults	HAPE in children	HAPE in adults	Reference
Tibet, 4550 m	464 (0–15 years)	5355	34%	38.2%	1.5%	1.27%	(Wu, 1994)
Colorado, 2835 m	558 (9–14 years)	None	28%*†	8%†	None	N/A	(Theis *et al.*, 1993; Honigman *et al.*, 1993)
Colorado, 3488 m	23 (3–36 months)	45	22%	20%	None	None	(Yaron *et al.*, 1998)
Colorado, 3109 m	37 (3–36 months)	38	19%	24%	None	None	(Yaron *et al.*, 2002)
Putre, Chile, 3500 m	6 (6–48 months)	15	100%	27%	None	None	(Moraga *et al.*, 2002)
	10 (13–18 years)		50%				

*In this study a control group travelling to a sea-level location reported a 21% rate of symptoms using the same AMS scoring system.
† Ascent from 1600 m to 2835 m.

Headache, nausea, fatigue, anorexia, dizziness and sleep disturbance are rarely reported by children under 5 years, and these classic symptoms of AMS may easily be overlooked. In young children (less than 3 years of age), non-specific symptoms such as lethargy, food refusal, irritability (increased fussiness), decreased playfulness, difficulty sleeping and excessive crying may be the only indication of altitude illness. As noted above, travel to any new environment may result in changes in patterns of sleep, appetite, activity and mood in young children. Differentiating such behavioural changes caused by travel alone from those caused by altitude illness can be difficult. Furthermore, all of these symptoms could be attributed to intercurrent illness, dietary indiscretion, intoxication (older children) or psychological factors associated with remote travel, but in the presence of such symptoms the possibility of altitude illness warrants urgent consideration of descent. Older children (> 8 years of age) can usually be relied upon to report symptoms in much the same way as adults (*see* Chapter 2).

For older children, a careful discussion of symptoms of altitude illness with both parents and children can aid early recognition of symptoms and prompt treatment.

Children from 3–8 years of age, and those with learning or communication difficulties, may be poor at describing their symptoms, making altitude illness difficult to recognize (Pollard *et al.*, 2001).

Prevention

Detailed recommendations for travel to altitude with children, adapted from an international consensus statement (Pollard *et al.*, 2001), are given later in this chapter. Little is known about altitude acclimatization in children, but one study that recorded the change in heart rate and arterial oxygen saturation of children aged 7–9 years and their adult parents during a slow graded ascent found that the children acclimatized as well as the adults (Tuggy *et al.*, 2000). Where altitude travel is undertaken with children, slow graded ascent is strongly advised, as has been suggested for adults (*see* Chapter 2), with the lowest possible sleeping altitude always selected in order to prevent altitude illness. Use of acetazolamide for AMS prophylaxis has not been studied in children, and in our view should not replace a cautious ascent schedule. Some organizations have recommended the large-scale use of acetazolamide for parties of children travelling to altitude, a practice which we find hard to justify. If acetazolamide is used in this way, informed parental and child consent should be sought.

Treatment

If there is a possibility that an ill child may have altitude illness then descent is recommended early, as it is difficult to assess severity, and the natural history of AMS in this age group has not been well characterized. Drug treatments for AMS could be considered as for adults, but using appropriate paediatric doses (*see* Box 4.1). Neither drugs nor treatment in a hyperbaric chamber have been subjected to controlled trials in children, but there is no reason to suggest that they will not be effective.

HACE in children

Only a very few cases of HACE in children have been reported (*see* table 2 in Pollard *et al.*, 2001), and there are no population-based studies that help in defining the incidence. Recognition and management are the same as described for adults (*see* Chapter 2). Early symptoms may be difficult to detect in children, particularly in those too young to communicate feelings of headache and nausea. Consequently, a high index of suspicion is required in order to recognize HACE in children. HACE should be managed by descent and administration of dexamethasone (*see* Box 4.1), acetazolamide and oxygen and treatment in a portable hyperbaric chamber.

HAPE in children

A large study of low altitude residents travelling in Tibet at 4550 m showed that HAPE occurred at the same frequency in adults as in children (1.27% and 1.51%, respectively) (Wu, 1994). It is uncertain whether this is true for all altitudes and rates of ascent. However, it is now well established that children normally resident at high altitude who return to a high altitude environment after a period at lower elevations are prone to re-entry pulmonary oedema (Marticorena *et al.*, 1964; Menon, 1965; Scoggin *et al.*, 1977; Hultgren and Marticorena, 1978; Fasules *et al.*, 1985; Hultgren, 1997), and develop a marked rise in their pulmonary artery pressure on exposure to hypoxia (Fasules *et al.*, 1985).

More than 290 cases of HAPE in children have been reported, although many of these were in high altitude residents who became unwell during

Box 4.1: Treatment of altitude illness in children

Acute mountain sickness
Mild
1 Rest (stop further ascent) or preferably descend until symptoms cease (particularly with younger children).
2 Symptomatic treatment, such as analgesics (paracetamol/acetaminophen 12 mg/kg po 6-hourly). Aspirin should be avoided in children because of the association with Reye's syndrome.

Moderate (worsening symptoms of AMS despite rest and symptomatic treatment)
1 Descent.
2 Oxygen.
3 Acetazolamide 2.5 mg/kg/dose po 8- to 12-hourly (maximum 250 mg per dose).
4 Dexamethasone 0.15 mg/kg/dose po 6-hourly.
5 Hyperbaric chamber (only used to facilitate descent, which should be undertaken as soon as possible).
6 Symptomatic treatment, such as analgesics (paracetamol/acetaminophen 12 mg/kg po 6-hourly). Use of aspirin is not recommended in young children, due to the association with Reye's syndrome.

High altitude pulmonary oedema
1 Descent.
2 Sit upright.
3 Oxygen.
4 Nifedipine 0.5 mg/kg/dose po 8-hourly (maximum 20 mg for capsules and 40 mg for tablets, slow-release preparation is preferred). Nifedipine is only necessary in those rare cases when response to oxygen and/or descent is unsatisfactory.
5 Use of dexamethasone should be considered because of associated HACE.
6 Hyperbaric chamber (only used to facilitate descent, which should be undertaken as soon as possible).

High altitude cerebral oedema
1 Descent.
2 Oxygen.
3 Dexamethasone 0.15 mg/kg/dose po 6-hourly.
4 Hyperbaric chamber (only used to facilitate descent, which should be undertaken as soon as possible).

reascent (Pollard *et al.*, 2001). Other underlying conditions that may have increased the risk of HAPE in these children include absent left pulmonary artery, congenital heart disease with pulmonary hypertension, patent ductus arteriosus, atrial septal defect, recent surgery for congenital cardiac disease, cardiomyopathy, cystic fibrosis, adrenogenital syndrome with cortisol deficiency, hypoventilation syndrome or obstructive sleep apnoea (e.g. associated with Down syndrome), Arnold–Chiari malformation, myelomeningocoele, perinatal hypoxia, ex-prematurity and bronchopulmonary dysplasia (Sartori *et al.*, 1999; Durmowicz, 2001; Pollard *et al.*, 2001; Schoene, 2001).

The symptoms, signs and management of HAPE in children are the same as those described for adults. Children may fail to report the subjective feelings of dyspnoea, fatigue, reduced exercise tolerance and cough even when they have become apparent clinically. Descent is vital. HAPE may be more likely to develop in children who are suffering from viral respiratory illnesses (Durmowicz *et al.*, 1997) shortly before or during ascent, and extra caution is required in this situation. Again no controlled trials of drug treatment have been performed in children, but in life-threatening situations paediatric doses should be used (*see* Box 4.1). To avoid systemic hypotension, sublingual nifedipine is best avoided.

Chronic altitude exposure in childhood

For the newborn at sea level, the increase in oxygen tension from the first breath initiates closure of the ductus arteriosus and drives a fall in pulmonary vascular resistance, thus reducing pulmonary arterial pressure. Oxygen saturations are lower in newborns at altitude than at sea level, and tend to drop during the first week of life and during sleep (Niermeyer *et al.*, 1993). It has been postulated that this may result from persistence of periodic breathing that is observed in infants at high altitude (Kelly *et al.*, 1985; Niermeyer *et al.*, 2001). Then, mean oxygen saturations steadily increase with age during childhood (data from 3800–4200 m in Tibet) during the first 10 years (Beall, 2000). Lower saturations have been noted in lowlanders at altitude (Han Chinese) than in native highlanders in Tibet, particularly during sleep, and are dependent on altitude (Niermeyer *et al.*, 1995). As a result of the hypoxia, the normal fall in pulmonary arterial pressure after birth may be delayed by several days or fail to occur at all, but these effects may be overcome by the administration of supplemental oxygen (Sime *et al.*, 1963; Niermeyer *et al.*, 1993), which is now routine at 3100 m in Leadville, Colorado (Niermeyer *et al.*, 1995, 2001). A further effect of the altitude hypoxia is failure of successful ductal occlusion, resulting in a higher incidence of patent ductus arteriosus noted in altitude residents of Cerro de Pasco (4330 m) compared with sea-level residents (0.74% and 0.05%, respectively) (Gamboa *et al.*, 1972). In Qinghai Province in China, 5% of children have an atrial septal defect or patent ductus arteriosus at 4500 m (Miao *et al.*, 1988). There was also a twofold increase in the incidence of neonatal hyperbilirubinaemia in another study at 3100 m in Colorado, which was thought to be due to increased bilirubin production (as a result of the increased haematocrit) and delayed bilirubin excretion.

Growth, puberty and menarche are delayed at high altitude. Birth weight is reduced at altitude starting from 1500 m (Yip, 1987), and there is significant postnatal growth retardation (Niermeyer *et al.*, 2001) that is partly due to the lower birth weight (Yip *et al.*, 1988). European girls (born at low altitude) living at altitude in La Paz (3600 m) reach menarche nearly two years later than European girls living at low altitude in Bolivia (Greksa, 1990). Menarche is much later in native highlanders in the Himalaya (16.8 years in one study) (Weitz *et al.*, 1978). The growth of low altitude children who are briefly exposed to altitude hypoxia is unlikely to be significantly affected, and any effect would probably be transient. Some climbers on expeditions to high altitude notice the development of transverse nail ridges coinciding with the time spent at altitude. This is probably a result of hypoxic and hypothermic slowing of nail growth. Exposure lasting for several months could reduce growth velocity in children, although there have been no studies of this. It is unclear whether any reduction in growth velocity could be counteracted by catch-up growth back at sea level following exposure.

The influence of prolonged exposure to altitude hypoxia on the developing brain is unknown.

Symptomatic high altitude pulmonary hypertension

Symptomatic high altitude pulmonary hypertension (SHAPH) includes acute exacerbations of pulmonary hypertension, as well as the syndrome of subacute infantile mountain sickness (SIMS) or high altitude heart disease that occurs in infants (under 1 year of age) after a prolonged stay (over 1 month) at altitudes over 3000 m (Wu and Liu, 1955; Khoury and Hawes, 1963; Sui et al., 1988; Wu, 1994; Pollard et al., 2001). Acute increases in pulmonary artery pressure have been observed in infants living at or travelling to high altitude in association with intercurrent viral infections (Susan Niermeyer, unpublished observation). Treatment of this condition focuses on oxygen administration and descent. The subacute form of SHAPH presents as right heart failure secondary to hypoxic pulmonary hypertension within a few months of birth at high altitude, or after arrival at high altitude from sea level. Many cases have been described in Tibet where those affected are infants of lowland Han Chinese origin (Wu, 1994). Right ventricular hypertrophy and muscularization of peripheral pulmonary arterioles are typical. Prevalence is 0.47% at 2261–2808 m and 0.96% at 3050–5188 m. Presentation is with signs and symptoms of heart failure, namely dyspnoea, cyanosis, cough, poor feeding, sweating, sleeplessness, irritability, hepatomegaly, facial oedema and oliguria. Mortality in hospitalized infants is 15% (Wu, 1994). Treatment of subacute SHAPH is directed at control of congestive cardiac failure and reversal of pulmonary hypertension by administration of oxygen, pharmacological diuresis and urgent descent.

Prolonged altitude travel for infants may expose them to a risk of SHAPH. Parents may well want to avoid this risk, but the minimum safe lengths of altitude exposure are unknown. Where it is necessary for infants to spend prolonged periods at high altitude, parents should be alerted to the possibility of SHAPH and arrangements for cardiological observation should be made. This condition may also rarely occur in older children and adults.

Children who are at obvious risk from hypoxic pulmonary hypertension (children with hypoxic lung disease, congenital heart disease, and children born prematurely) should avoid altitude exposure wherever possible, as this may precipitate a pulmonary hypertensive crisis.

Box **4.2:** Children and altitude illness

- Diagnosis is difficult.

- Non-specific symptoms predominate.

- If in doubt, descend until symptoms resolve.

Sudden infant death syndrome

One study has shown that there is a good correlation between the risk of sudden infant death syndrome (SIDS) and altitude exposure up to 1500 m (Getts and Hill, 1982). This study did not examine populations living above 1500 m, but it is possible that chronic altitude hypoxia above this height increases the risk of SIDS and might further support an argument against taking infants to high altitudes. However, another study failed to confirm this association (Barkin *et al.*, 1981). There is certainly a well-documented increase in infant mortality among high altitude residents. Studies of breathing patterns in infants at altitude have noted a prolongation of normal neonatal periodic breathing and desaturations in sleep in Denver, Colorado (1610 m), suggesting that exposure to altitude may interfere with the normal respiratory adaptation that occurs following birth (Niermeyer, 1997; Parkins *et al.*, 1998).

As at sea level, the risk of SIDS is reduced by putting the baby down to sleep supine, and by avoiding exposure of the infant to cigarette smoke (Kohlendorfer *et al.*, 1998; Wisborg *et al.*, 2000).

An international consensus statement on special considerations for ascent to altitude with children (reproduced with permission from Pollard *et al.*, 2001)

General comments

1   There are no data on safe absolute altitudes for ascent in children.

2   The risk of acute altitude illness is for ascents above around 2500 m, particularly sleeping above 2500 m.

3   Intercurrent illness might increase the risk of altitude illness.

4   The effects of longer-term (weeks) exposure to altitude hypoxia on over-all growth and brain and cardiopulmonary development are unknown.

Location of travel

Travel to high altitude in mountain and ski resorts in industrialized countries with easy and rapid access to medical care should be considered differently from remote travel in isolated mountain ranges and areas without access to a high level of medical sophistication.

1   Most mountain tourist sites and ski resorts in industrialized countries are located at or below about 3000 m, and the majority of travellers to these sites will sleep at about 3000 m or less. Acute mountain sickness is common at this altitude, and there is probably a small risk of serious altitude illness. Once recognized, altitude illness is effectively managed with oxygen and/or descent in most cases. Ascents during tourist activities (cable car rides, travel on mountain roads and ski trips) higher than the resort location, to about 4000 m, are usually brief (hours) and probably carry minimal additional risk. Longer trips above 3000 m on foot or horseback should be undertaken with slow, graded and cautious ascent to reduce the possibility of altitude illness.

2   Ascents made in remote mountain locations without rapid access to medical care should be undertaken with greater caution. Ascents with sleeping altitudes at or below 3000 m carry a low risk of serious altitude illness, but if HAPE or HACE occur, management can be more difficult than in developed areas. Higher ascents in this context should be undertaken with slow graded ascent, rest (acclimatization) days and careful emergency planning.

Age of the child

1   Altitude illness is particularly difficult to recognize in preverbal children (< 3 years), who cannot report classic symptoms of mountain

sickness. Similarly, some children from 3–8 years of age may be good at reporting symptoms, but extra caution is required for the younger children in this age range, and children with learning difficulties who will have difficulty expressing their experience of symptoms of acute altitude illness. Older children (> 8 years) have usually reached the developmental level necessary to report these symptoms.

2   Many preverbal children travel to resorts at 3000 m in North American mountain ranges without complications, but extra caution is required for higher ascents and for ascents in remote areas.

3   For infants in the first few weeks and months of life, there may be some additional theoretical concerns that exposure to over 2500 m for more than a few hours may affect normal respiratory patterns (Parkins *et al.*, 1998).

Length of altitude exposure

1   Ascents higher than 3000 m that are prolonged (> 1 day) or require sleeping above 3000 m increase the risk of acute mountain sickness and should be undertaken cautiously with slow graded ascent, built-in rest days and emergency planning.

2   In circumstances where the child is travelling above 2500 m altitude because of parental occupation *and* prolonged altitude residence is anticipated, slow graded ascent as described earlier should be undertaken. For infants (< 1 year) in families that are planning to reside permanently at altitude, some authorities recommend delaying ascent to altitude until beyond the first year of life because of the slight risk of SHAPH (*see* page 50) above 3000 m. This is usually impractical if parental separation is to be avoided. Therefore, after a careful physical examination before ascent and initial acclimatization to high altitude, the infant should be monitored closely with regard to growth percentiles. Pulse oximetry may be useful, especially during sleep, and the ECG should be monitored periodically for the development of right ventricular hypertrophy.

Cold, sun and the child at altitude

Cold exposure is a particular risk for children on mountains. The increased risk is due to a combination of large surface area acting as a heat exchanger, excessive energy expenditure or low energy production (the sleeping carried child), and failure to wear adequate clothing (preverbal children may not complain, and older children may dress inappropriately for a number of reasons). Particular attention should be paid to adequate insulation of the head and extremities, and a windproof outer layer is important. A child who is being carried is not generating heat, and at low ambient temperatures they will need extra layers of clothing even when the adult who is carrying them is comfortably warm. Frostbite of the extremities while a child is being carried (during walking or skiing) is a recognized hazard (unpublished observations cited in Pollard *et al.*, 2001), and death from hypothermia has been known to occur.

Box 4.3: Cold

- Windproof

- Waterproof

- Insulate

The dangers of ultraviolet radiation should be constantly considered. UVA + UVB sunblock creams (SPF $\geq$ 30, applied before exposure to sun), hats and long-sleeved clothing should always be used. Burning may occur even on cloudy days, especially in snow. Infants are especially vulnerable. Goggles are required to prevent snowblindness, and can be difficult to keep on unwilling young children. Overheating may also occur, particularly on sunny days and during glacier travel.

Box 4.4: Sunburn and snowblindness

- Cover up with long-sleeved tops and long trousers

- Use sunblock on all exposed skin

- Wear goggles

Fluid balance and the child at altitude

Adequate fluid intake in a dry altitude environment is important for all ages (*see* Table 4.2). Children may need encouragement to ensure they drink enough to meet the increase in requirements. Diarrhoeal illnesses are common during travel to many of the remote mountain regions of the world, and are considered in Chapter 8.

Table 4.2: Normal minimum maintenance fluid requirements for children at sea level in a temperate climate

Weight (kg)	Total fluid/24 hours (ml)	Weight (kg)	Total fluid/24 hours (ml)
4	480–600	18	1440
6	600–720	20	1560
8	800	30	1680
10	960	40	1920
12	1080	50	2160
14	1200	60	2280
16	1320	70	2400

Emotions and children at altitude

The family expedition or school trip to a mountain environment can generate emotional dilemmas for parents and children. Children may find the experience stressful, and parents will find the everyday problems of caring for children magnified by the loss of comforts such as hot water and disposable nappies. Faced with iodinated water to drink and local food to eat, infants and young children may refuse food, causing parental anxiety and conflict. Infants can become dehydrated through refusal to drink. Young children usually have a short attention span and easily become bored after travelling a relatively short distance. A stimulating itinerary should therefore be carefully chosen. Finally, parents may find it difficult to be rational about the management of their own sick or injured child when in a remote environment.

Preparation for altitude travel with children

Travelling to remote mountain wildernesses with children requires special considerations regardless of the altitude. Careful planning to ensure flexibility, particularly during ascent, is important to allow time for intercurrent illnesses, acclimatization and even time to wash clothes. Where children are to be carried, itineraries depend on the stamina of the adult doing the carrying. Local porters will often be prepared to carry children. Cautious estimates for distances walked per day by children of different ages have been suggested (2–3 years, 0.5–2 miles; 4–6 years, 3–5 miles; 7–9 years, 5–7 miles; 10–13 years, 8–10 miles; 14–18 years, adult distances). Some children may be accustomed to longer distances (Gentile and Kennedy, 1991).

The mountain environment may be particularly hazardous to the young child who is less aware of potentially dangerous situations and may not have the necessary motor or hand–eye co-ordination skills to escape harm. Adequate supervision should be planned, particularly in school groups, and carers should have considered rescue arrangements. A general first-aid course may help to avoid preventable tragedy.

Medical and surgical complications are discussed in Chapter 9. Clearly, appropriate paediatric doses of drugs should be checked by a doctor advising any group that includes children. A careful medical history taken prior to departure is necessary to document important conditions, including cardiovascular, pulmonary or allergic disorders.

Box 4.5: Preparation for a trek with children

- Be realistic about the objective.

- Be realistic about the distances which can be covered each day.

- Plan evacuation and rescue.

- Train the parents in first aid.

References and further reading

Barkin RM, Hartley MR and Brooks JG (1981) Influence of high altitude on sudden infant death syndrome. *Pediatrics*. **68**: 981–2.

Bärtsch P (1994) Going to high altitude with children. *Newsletter Int Soc Mountain Med*. **4**: 2–3.

Beall CM (2000) Oxygen saturation increases during childhood and decreases during adulthood among high altitude native Tibetians residing at 3800–4200 m. *High Alt Med Biol*. **1**: 25–32.

Durmowicz AG (2001) Pulmonary edema in 6 children with Down syndrome during travel to moderate altitudes. *Pediatrics*. **108**: 443–7.

Durmowicz AG, Noordeweir E and Nicholas R (1997) Inflammatory processes may predispose children to high altitude pulmonary edema. *J Pediatr*. **130**: 838–40.

Fasules J, Wiggins J and Wolfe R (1985) Increased lung vasoreactivity in children from Leadville, Colorado, after recovery from high altitude pulmonary oedema. *Circulation*. **72**: 957–62.

Gamboa R, Marticorena E and Penaloza D (1972) The ductus arteriosus in the newborn infant at high altitude. *Vasa*. **1**: 192–5.

Gentile DA and Kennedy BC (1991) Wilderness medicine for children. *Pediatrics*. **88**: 967–81.

Getts AG and Hill HF (1982) Sudden infant death syndrome: incidence at various altitudes. *Dev Med Child Neurol*. **24**: 61–8.

Greksa LP (1990) Age of menarche in Bolivian girls of European and Aymara ancestry. *Ann Hum Biol*. **17**: 49–53.

Honigman B, Theis MK, Koziol-McLain J *et al*. (1993) Acute mountain sickness in a general tourist population at moderate altitudes. *Ann Intern Med*. **118**(8): 587–92.

Hultgren H (1997) High altitude pulmonary edema. In: H Hultgren (ed.) *High Altitude Medicine*. Hultgren Publications, Stanford, CA.

Hultgren H and Marticorena E (1978) High altitude pulmonary oedema: epidemiologic observations in Peru. *Chest*. **74**: 372–6.

Jean D (1994) Child and altitude. *Newsletter Int Soc Mountain Med.* **4**: 3–4.

Kelly DH, Stellwagen LM, Kaitz E *et al.* (1985) Apnea and periodic breathing in normal full-term infants during the first twelve months. *Pediatr Pulmonol.* **1**: 215–19.

Khoury GH and Hawes CR (1963) Primary pulmonary hypertension in children living at high altitude. *J Pediatr.* **62**: 177–85.

Kohlendorfer U, Kiechl S and Sperl W (1998) Living at high altitude and risk of sudden infant death syndrome. *Arch Dis Child.* **79**: 506–9.

Leibson C, Brown M, Thibodeau S *et al.* (1988) Neonatal hyperbilirubinemia at high altitude. *Am J Dis Child.* **143**: 983–7.

Maggiorini M, Bühler B, Walter M *et al.* (1990) Prevalence of acute mountain sickness in the Swiss Alps. *BMJ.* **301**: 853–5.

Marticorena E, Tapia FA, Dyer J *et al.* (1964) Pulmonary edema by ascending to high altitudes. *Dis Chest.* **45**: 273.

Menon ND (1965) High altitude pulmonary edema: a clinical study. *NEJM.* **273**: 66–73.

Miao CY, Zuberbuhler JS and Zuberbuhler JR (1988) Prevalence of congenital cardiac anomalies at high altitude. *J Am Coll Cardiol.* **12**: 224–8.

Moraga FA, Osorio JD and Vargas ME (2002) Acute mountain sickness in tourists with children at Lake Chungara (4400 m) in northern Chile. *Wild Environ Med.* **13**: 31–5.

Niermeyer S (1997) The newborn at high altitude: cardiopulmonary function. In: JR Sutton, CS Houston and G Coates (eds) *Hypoxia and the Brain.* Queen City Printers, Burlington, VT.

Niermeyer S, Shaffer EM, Thilo E *et al.* (1993) Arterial oxygenation and pulmonary arterial pressure in healthy neonates and infants at high altitude. *J Pediatr.* **123**: 767–72.

Niermeyer S, Yang P, Shanmina *et al.* (1995) Arterial oxygen saturation in Tibetan and Han infants born in Lhasa, Tibet. *NEJM.* **333**: 1248–52.

Niermeyer S, Zamudio S and Moore LG (2001) The people. In: TF Hornbein and RB Schoene (eds) *High Altitude: an exploration of human adaptation.* Marcel Dekker Inc, New York, pp. 43–100.

Parkins KJ, Poets CF, O'Brien LM *et al.* (1998) Effect of exposure to 15% oxygen on breathing patterns and oxygen saturation in infants: interventional study. *BMJ.* **316**: 887–91.

Pollard AJ, Murdoch DR and Bärtsch P (1998) Children in the mountains. *BMJ.* **316**: 874–5.

Pollard AJ, Niermeyer S, Barry P *et al.* (2001) Children at high altitude: an international consensus statement by an ad hoc committee of the International Society for Mountain Medicine. *High Alt Med Biol.* **2**: 389–403.

Sartori C, Allemann Y, Trueb L *et al.* (1999) Augmented vasoreactivity in adult life associated with perinatal vascular insult. *Lancet.* **353**: 2205–7.

Schoene RB (2001) Fatal high altitude pulmonary edema associated with absence of the left pulmonary artery. *High Alt Med Biol.* **2**: 405–6.

Scoggin CH, Hyers TM, Reeves JT *et al.* (1977) High altitude pulmonary edema in the children and young adults of Leadville, Colorado. *NEJM.* **297**: 1269–72.

Sime F, Banchero N, Penaloza D *et al.* (1963) Pulmonary hypertension in children born and living at high altitudes. *Am J Cardiol.* **11**: 143–9.

Sui GJ, Liu YH, Cheng XS *et al.* (1988) Subacute infantile mountain sickness. *J Pathol.* **155**: 161–70.

Theis MK, Honigman B, Yip R *et al.* (1993) Acute mountain sickness in children at 2835 meters. *Am J Dis Child.* **147**: 143–5.

Tuggy ML, Sarjeant P, Litch JA *et al.* (2000) Comparison of acclimatization to high altitude between genetically related adults and children. *Wild Environ Med.* **11**: 292–5.

Weitz CA, Pawson IG, Wetz MW *et al.* (1978) Cultural factors affecting the demographic structures of a high altitude Nepalese population. *Soc Biol.* **25**: 179–95.

Wisborg K, Kesmodel U, Henriksen TB *et al.* (2000) A prospective study of smoking during pregnancy and SIDS. *Arch Dis Child.* **83**: 203–6.

Wu DC and Liu YR (1955) High altitude heart disease. *Chin J Pediat.* **6**: 348–50.

Wu T (1994) Children on the Tibetan Plateau. *Newsletter Int Soc Mountain Med.* **4**: 5–7.

Wu TY (1983) An investigation of high altitude heart disease. *Chin Nat J Med.* **67**: 90–2.

Yaron M, Waldman N, Niermeyer S *et al.* (1997) The diagnosis of acute mountain sickness in pre-verbal children. In: CS Houston and G Coates (eds) *Hypoxia: women at altitude.* Queen City Printers, Burlington, VT.

Yaron M, Waldman N, Niermeyer S *et al.* (1998) The diagnosis of acute mountain sickness in preverbal children. *Arch Pediatr Adolesc Med.* **152**: 683–7.

Yaron M, Niermeyer S, Lindgren KN *et al.* (2002) Evaluation of diagnostic criteria and incidence of acute mountain sickness in preverbal children. *Wild Environ Med.* **13**: 21–6.

Yip R (1987) Altitude and birthweight. *J Pediatr.* **111**: 869–76.

Yip R, Binkin N and Trowbridge FL (1988) Altitude and childhood growth. *J Pediatr.* **113**: 486–9.

5

Cold and heat related conditions

Hypothermia

Hypothermia is defined as a reduction in the core temperature to below 35°C. Acute hypothermia follows a sudden drop in body temperature over minutes to hours, as occurs with immersion in cold water or a sudden climatic change. Subacute or chronic hypothermia results from a more gradual drop in core temperature over hours to days. In a mountain environment this typically occurs in the setting of inadequate clothing or shelter. Hypothermia is considered mild if the core temperature is between 32°C and 35°C, while core temperatures less than 32°C represent severe hypothermia. Children and lean young men are at particular risk.

Clinical features

Mild hypothermia
Mild hypothermia manifests as fine motor inco-ordination and loss of judgement in an otherwise fully conscious individual. Shivering is usually present, and a stumbling gait may develop.

Severe hypothermia
Altered mental status becomes profound as the core temperature drops below 32°C, with deteriorating memory, apathy and poor decision making, progressing to coma. Speech is often slurred. Shivering stops below 30°C core temperature, pupils may be fixed and dilated, the body will be cold to touch and the muscles become rigid. There may be profound bradycardia and depressed respiratory rate. The skin may be pale and oedematous. Hypoglycaemia is common. The patient may appear dead,

although this should not be presumed unless there is no response to rewarming. Asystole may occur. Ventricular fibrillation may be precipitated by attempts to move or even resuscitate the victim, particularly if the core temperature is below 28°C. The development of ataxia in a cold-exposed individual suggests hypothermia or (at high altitude) high altitude cerebral oedema.

Table 5.1: Hypothermia

Rectal temperature (°C)	Clinical features
37	Normal (37.6°C is normal rectal temperature)
36	Tachycardia and increase in metabolic rate
35	Tachycardia, maximal shivering, vasoconstriction and mild confusion
33	Severe confusion, apathy and ataxia, shivering
31–2	Shivering ceases, stupor
28–30	Bradycardia, hypoventilation, dilated pupils, coma, ventricular fibrillation
25–7	Loss of all tendon reflexes, voluntary movements and response to pain
24	Loss of blood pressure and severe bradycardia
23	Loss of corneal reflexes
20	Asystole (reversible)

Management

The management of hypothermia is outlined in Figure 5.1. The principles of management include:

1   prevention of further heat loss

2   restoration of body temperature to normal

3   supportive care to facilitate principles 1 and 2

4   treatment of the underlying condition (trauma, cardiac event, hypoglycaemia, etc.).

A low-reading thermometer is required to measure case temperature in the hypothermic casualty, as ordinary thermometers will only read down to 34°C.

Mild hypothermia (32–35°C)

Further heat loss should be prevented by removal from the cold environment and protecting from wet, wind and cold. Improving insulation by replacing wet clothes, covering the head and extremities and insulating from the ground will reduce heat loss further. This may be all that is needed in order to allow gradual rewarming. External heat sources such as hot packs and hot-water bottles may be helpful in a remote setting, but should not be applied directly to the skin because of the risk of burning. Active external warming with hot packs applied to the axillae, groin, neck (over the carotids) and chest are most efficient at raising core temperature, and are less likely to induce peripheral vasodilation and circulatory collapse. Zipping two sleeping bags together and placing the patient inside with one or two normothermic individuals is a useful method for applying an external heat source. Drinking warm sweet fluids will add to warming and correct hypoglycaemia. Administration of warm inspired oxygen may aid rewarming, but will not usually be possible in a mountain environment. Warmed intravenous fluids should not be given in the hope of raising body temperature, as the volume required to do this is very large. However, if intravenous fluids are given, they should be warmed to prevent further cooling of the body.

Severe hypothermia (< 32°C)

Individuals with severe hypothermia must be handled as gently as possible and remain in a horizontal position because of the risk of provoking ventricular fibrillation by moving, jarring, upright position or even inappropriate resuscitation. Asystole is very difficult to diagnose in the severely hypothermic casualty in the field, because of the victim's cold tissues and the rescuer's vasoconstricted cold fingers which make palpation of the arterial pulse difficult. The profound bradycardia in severe hypothermia may be adequate for cerebral metabolism, but inappropriate attempts at resuscitation and cardiac massage may provoke ventricular fibrillation which, without cardiopulmonary resuscitation (CPR), will not sustain cerebral perfusion. Profound bradycardia is not an indication for CPR in severe hypothermia. In less remote areas where a mountain rescue team is at hand, defibrillation equipment may be available on the mountainside and active CPR is indicated for ventricular fibrillation (carotid pulse will be lacking in this case). The ventricular fibrillation encountered in hypothermia may be unresponsive to usual advanced management (DC shock and medications), at least prior to rewarming the patient to 30°C (Resuscitation Council (UK), 1996).

In the pulseless hypothermic individual, CPR (*see* Chapter 9) should only be commenced where there is no pulsation after one minute of palpation of the carotid artery **and** resuscitation can be continued until evacuation (Weinberg, 1993; Lloyd, 1994; Durrer and Brugger, 1997). Some authorities recommend that CPR is only commenced if these criteria are satisfied **and** cardiac arrest has been observed (or is likely to have occurred within the previous two hours) (Handley *et al.*, 1993; Snadden, 1993). However, in most cases the time of cardiopulmonary arrest is unknown and active management should be undertaken. It is unrealistic to undertake CPR during a stretcher evacuation in any case in severe hypothermia. Even when CPR is delayed until arrival in hospital and the victim is asystolic, survival may be possible with advanced support and rewarming techniques in an intensive care unit (ICU). In hypothermia the tissues are stiffer and there is more resistance to chest compression and assisted ventilation.

Diagnosis of irreversible hypothermia is a problem in the field. Survival has been possible in therapeutic hypothermia down to core temperatures of just 9°C (15°C in accidental hypothermia). Irreversible hypothermia is probable if there is asystole, the chest is not compressible and the abdominal muscles are not kneadable or the core temperature is below 9°C (Durrer and Brugger, 1997). Serum potassium greater than 12 mmol/l seems to be incompatible with survival (Durrer and Brugger, 1997). New recommendations for mountain rescue teams have been published recently (Durrer *et al.*, 2003) which provide a consensus about the approach to the hypothermic victim where there is specific expertise and medical equipment available by the rescue doctor.

When in a remote wilderness location, commencing CPR with no hope of evacuation within a few hours is likely to exhaust those administering it and put their own lives at risk. If evacuation is impossible, CPR should only be commenced in the field when it can be continued until the victim has been rewarmed. This may take many hours in the field (see below).

Thermal clothing and other insulating layers (e.g. sleeping bag) are useful for heat retention. Since most heat loss is by conduction or convection rather than radiation, aluminium foil blankets are less useful and may be unmanageable in high winds. Wet clothes should not be removed until shelter is reached (an ambient temperature of 25°C is ideal, but unlikely to be achieved in the field), when they should be gently cut away and changed for dry clothes. Changing wet clothes could precipitate venticular fibrillation or further cooling and hypotension, and if shelter cannot be reached the wet clothes should be left and covered with an improvised vapour barrier. Oxygen should be administered, if available. Normally the patient should be evacuated as soon as possible after initial attempts to reverse heat loss, as it is both difficult and dangerous to try to adequately rewarm a severely hypothermic patient in the field. Where evacuation is impossible, rewarming must be undertaken in the field. This is hazardous because of the risk of ventricular fibrillation, and should not be undertaken lightly. The victim should be placed in the recovery position to protect the airway, handled gently and maintained in a horizontal position.

There is a risk of peripheral vasodilation and hypovolaemic shock when active external warming is used. External heat sources such as hot packs and hot-water bottles should only be placed on the chest, axillae, groin and neck to produce warming, and are used more commonly than immersion in water at 40°C, which is more likely to precipitate generalized vasodilation. Rewarming with hot packs is a slow process. A maximal rate of 0.5–1°C per hour may be achieved using hot packs (Weinberg, 1993). Oxygen/air heaters designed for field use are the only practical active internal warming method during field evacuation, but are rarely available. Warmed intravenous fluids or enteral fluids via a nasogastric tube may be helpful but are also not without hazard. Other rewarming methods are not practical in the field.

Wherever possible, after preventing further heat loss by insulating with clothing, slow rewarming should be undertaken in an intensive-care unit. Use of warmed inspired ventilator gases, extracorporeal warming of blood, and pleural or peritoneal lavage all have their advocates. Using these techniques, rates of rewarming of up to 2.5°C per hour may be achieved. Again, there is a risk of ventricular fibrillation, but this is less than the risk with slower external rewarming.

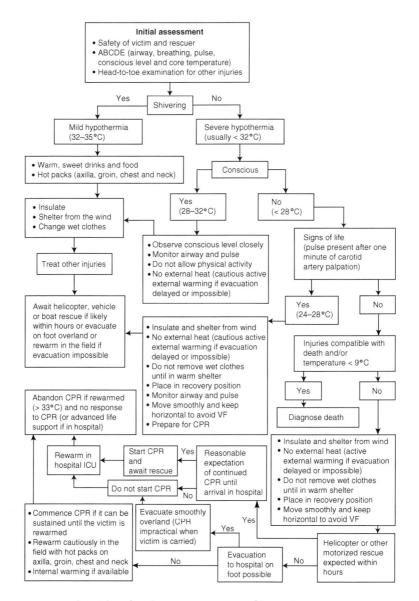

Figure 5.1: Algorithm for the management of hypothermia. Core temperatures (low-reading thermometer) are included for information, but are not usually available (Handley *et al.*, 1993; Snadden, 1993; Weinberg, 1993; Hodkin *et al.*, 1994; Lloyd, 1994; Resuscitation Council (UK), 1996; Durrer and Brugger, 1997).

Box 5.1: Rules for management of hypothermia

- Prevent it by adequate insulation, waterproof and windproof outer layers of clothing

Mild

- Rewarm by sharing body heat and insulating from heat loss
- Correct hypoglycaemia

Severe

- Handle carefully because of risk of cardiac arrhythmia
- Rewarm slowly, preferably after evacuation

Avalanche

Avalanche victims usually die from asphyxia rather than hypothermia, and their survival chances depend on the time taken for rescue (Falk *et al.*, 1994). The snow cover insulates the buried victim and the onset of hypothermia is slow (3°C per hour maximum). Survival is 92% at 15 minutes, 30% at 35 minutes and only a few per cent at 130 minutes. About one-third of avalanche victims manage to create an air pocket during the avalanche, and they have a reasonable chance of surviving to 90 minutes. Decisions regarding resuscitation depend on the burial time, presence of an air pocket, obstruction of the airway by snow, core temperature, presence of a pulse and other injuries (Brugger *et al.*, 1996, 2001; Brugger and Durrer, 2002). The algorithm shown in Figure 5.2 is a suggested management plan for avalanche victims. The safety precautions for rescuers entering avalanche terrain must be maintained at all times. Recommendations for the management of avalanche casualties by fully equipped rescue teams are given by Brugger and Durrer (2002).

Frostbite

Frostbite occurs at temperatures below 0°C and is due to freezing with consequent death of tissues. The risk of frostbite depends on the environmental temperature, the windchill factor (Wilson and Goldman, 1970)

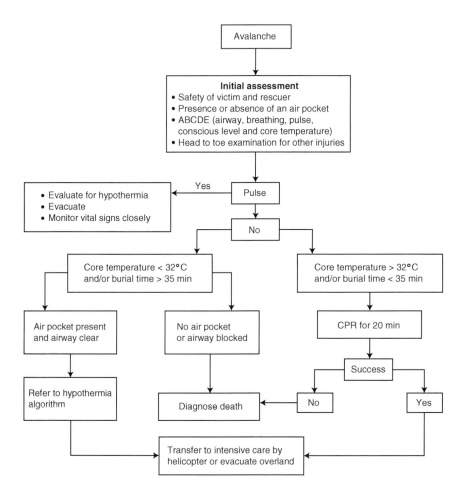

Figure 5.2: Management of avalanche casualties (Falk *et al.*, 1994; Brugger *et al.*, 1996, 2001; Durrer and Brugger, 1997; Brugger and Durrer, 2002).

and the length of exposure. Frostbite is more likely to occur in the presence of high winds, high altitude, contact with heat-conductive materials such as metal (e.g. spectacle frames, seats) and water, dehydration, hypovolaemia, tobacco use and any other factors that reduce blood supply to the extremities (e.g. ill-fitting boots, rings on fingers, and pre-existing vascular disease, including Raynaud's syndrome).

Clinical features

Frostbite can affect any area, but is especially common on the hands and feet. It may also affect the face (nose, chin, earlobes, cheeks, lips) and buttocks/perineum (from sitting on metallic seats).

Frost-nip

The skin becomes white and loses sensation, but remains viable. On rewarming, the skin becomes hyperaemic and paraesthetic and recovers completely. Complete return of sensation may take weeks.

Superficial frostbite

Both skin and subcutaneous tissues are involved. The skin is initially pale and cold, but the underlying deep tissues remain undamaged. Blisters usually develop within one to two days and resolve to form a black carapace. The carapace is denervated and painless and separates from viable tissue along a sharp line of demarcation after several weeks.

Deep frostbite

Deeper structures are affected, including muscle, tendons and occasionally bone. The affected part is insensitive and hard. Blisters develop and eventually gangrene with inevitable tissue loss.

Using experience of frostbite in the French Alps, Cauchy *et al.* (2001) have proposed a new classification of frostbite severity at day 0 in four stages based on a combination of clinical and bone-scan information. First-degree frostbite is likely to lead to recovery, second-degree frostbite will result in soft tissue amputation, third-degree frostbite leads to bone amputation, and fourth-degree frostbite leads to amputation of a large area.

Prevention

Measures to prevent frostbite include retaining heat through adequate clothing (which insulates, and is waterproof and windproof), avoiding constriction of body parts with clothing or other items (especially avoid tight footwear), wearing mittens instead of gloves, staying dry, avoiding direct contact with heat-conductive materials, and maintaining hydration and an adequate caloric intake.

Management

The principles of management include:

1   treatment of associated hypothermia urgently

2   prevention of further damage to the skin

3   avoidance of re-freezing

4   rapid rewarming as soon as re-freezing can be avoided

5   prevention of infection

6   delayed surgery.

Prior to management of frostbite, any associated hypothermia should always be aggressively treated as described earlier in this chapter.

Further damage to the frostbitten limb should be prevented by careful and gentle handling of the affected limb, which should not be rubbed (including with snow or ice), beaten or overheated with external heat sources such as fires, as all of these may worsen the injury. The affected part must be sheltered from the wind and relieved of any other cofactors that might reduce blood supply (e.g. ill-fitting boots). Wet gloves and socks should be changed. Some authorities also recommend a single dose of aspirin to improve circulation in the field (assuming that there are no contraindications) (Syme, 2002).

Thawing in the field runs the risk of immediate and disastrous re-freezing and, ideally, rewarming and further management should take place in hospital. Evacuation is often easier if the extremities remain frozen (it is possible to walk with frozen toes, but it may be too painful once thawing has taken place). In some situations when evacuation is not immediately possible, rewarming in the field may be necessary using shared body heat. The affected limb is placed in a companion's armpit or groin for up to 10 minutes (Syme, 2002). At extreme altitude (> 5000 m) oxygen should be administered as soon as possible.

Rewarming should be undertaken within 48 hours of the onset of frostbite wherever possible. Once in a safe environment, preferably in hospital, the limb is rapidly rewarmed by placing in warm water (37°C) and thawing over 30 minutes. Slow rewarming should be avoided as it causes more tissue damage. Most authorities reserve the use of antibiotics for treatment only. Pain relief will be necessary once rewarming is undertaken, and opiates are often required. Vasodilators (e.g. nifedipine/reserpine) are recommended by some immediately before rewarming, and some have used them prophylactically, but their effectiveness is debatable. The fingers or toes should be loosely bandaged after rewarming, with plenty of padding between the digits. Movement of the digits should be encouraged, but the damaged tissues should not be used. This means that the

---

Box 5.2: Management of frostbite

Do not:
- Rub or beat

- Use an external heat source such as a fire or stove

- Allow re-freezing once thawed

- Submit to early amputations

- Rewarm a frostbitten part unless hypothermia has been treated first

Do:
- Rewarm rapidly, preferably in hospital and within 48 hours of the injury

- Give analgesia

- Encourage movement and avoid infection

- Delay surgery

---

individual will need a certain amount of assistance, especially with basic personal hygiene.

Once it has been rewarmed, the affected limb should be protected from trauma. Evacuation must be assisted, as extensive tissue damage will result from 'walking out' on a rewarmed frostbitten foot. Blisters are best left intact.

Subsequent management is best undertaken in hospital with careful removal of sloughing tissue in a whirlpool. Final surgical debridement should be delayed for up to three months unless infection prompts earlier intervention.

Sequelae of frostbite

Full recovery from frostbite may take up to a year. Once a person has suffered from frostbite, there is an increased chance of further cold injury to that digit, even with a lesser cold exposure than that which caused the initial insult. Mild cold exposure may result in pain or cracking of the skin. Some individuals have constant pain or loss of sensation which may never recover. Care is required following an episode of frostbite to avoid further damage (*see* Prevention, page 70).

Trench foot

Trench foot is the result of prolonged exposure of the lower extremities to temperatures between 0°C and 15°C, without freezing of tissues. Injury to soft tissues (especially peripheral nerves) occurs and may be irreversible. Affected limbs appear pale, pulseless and anaesthetic, and these features remain after rewarming. Risk factors include wet conditions, constrictive clothing and boots, hypothermia and immobility.

Typically, within one to two days of rewarming, hyperaemia of the affected limbs develops, associated with burning pain and the gradual return of sensation proximally. As perfusion increases, oedema and bullae may appear. Sensation usually recovers over several weeks, often associated with hyperhidrosis. Pulselessness after two days suggests severe deep injury and a high likelihood of significant tissue loss.

Prevention involves several basic measures.

1   Ensure that boots fit properly.

2   Avoid hypothermia.

3   Remove boots and socks at least twice daily, and dry and massage feet until circulation and sensation have returned. Put on socks that are dry (or as dry as possible).

4   Do not sleep in wet footgear.

5   Keep feet out of water and mud as much as possible.

6   Keep legs moving to stimulate circulation.

7   Observe carefully for numbness and tingling (the early symptoms of trench foot).

A number of other cold related conditions that affect the skin, particularly of the extremities, are well recognized. Perhaps the most common of these is Raynaud's syndrome, which may either occur in isolation or be associated with an underlying rheumatological disease such as systemic lupus erythematosus or scleroderma.

Chronic episodic severe vasoconstriction, often associated with cold exposure, leads to atrophic changes in the extremities of the digits.

Perniosis (chilblains) is characterized by localized tender inflammatory red or purple skin lesions that occur as an abnormal reaction to cold damp environments, and has been associated with river crossings (Price and Murdoch, 2001). Lesions occur in particular on the fingers, toes, heels, lower legs, thighs, nose and ears, and are more common in women. Perniosis often appears several hours after cold exposure and usually resolves over one to three weeks. Treatment is symptomatic, although nifedipine may reduce pain and resolution time.

Peripheral cyanosis (acrocyanosis) is very common in the extremities in cold conditions, but is not usually associated with an underlying pathological process.

Heat exhaustion and heat stroke

Huge variations in temperature are frequently observed in a mountain environment, particularly at high altitude. In the Western Cwm on Mount

Everest (6000–7000 m), the temperature in the sun may be over 30°C but can drop below freezing in minutes as the sun disappears behind the surrounding mountains. A degree of acclimatization occurs to both hot and cold temperatures. Acclimatization to a hot environment is achieved by increasing the maximum volume and decreasing the sodium content of sweat. For the unacclimatized individual from a temperate country, arrival in the tropics may precipitate heat exhaustion or heat stroke.

Heat exhaustion is usually associated with exercise in hot weather, and is the result of salt and water loss through sweating, inadequately replaced by oral intake. Early symptoms such as profuse sweating, dizziness, fatigue, myalgia, headache and lightheadedness may progress to hyperthermia (core temperature 38–40°C) and hypovolaemia. It is distinguished from heat stroke by the presence of essentially intact mentation and body temperature under 40°C. Treatment consists of shielding from the sun, fanning or cool sponging and oral rehydration. In severe cases, where facilities are available, careful electrolyte monitoring and intravenous rehydration should be undertaken.

In heat stroke, normal thermoregulatory mechanisms are lost and core body temperature rises above 41°C. This is a medical emergency. Although dehydration is not usually present initially, early symptoms are the same as for heat exhaustion. However, sweating ceases, the skin is hot to touch, and headache and gastrointestinal disturbance are prominent. Acute

---

Box 5.3:   Heat exhaustion and heat stroke

Heat exhaustion:
- is characterized by sweating, syncope, myalgia and fatigue

- is caused by dehydration and salt depletion

- is managed with rehydration and cooling.

Heat stroke:
- is hyperthermia with headache, central nervous system (CNS) disturbance and gastrointestinal disturbance

- treatment requires urgent skin surface cooling.

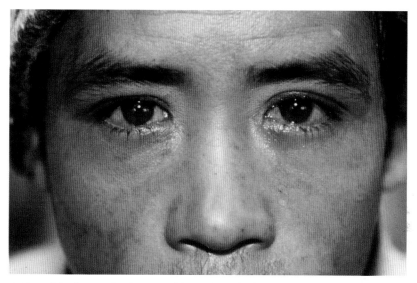

1 Snowblindness. A sherpa with conjunctivitis and lid oedema following glacier travel without goggles. (L Cook)

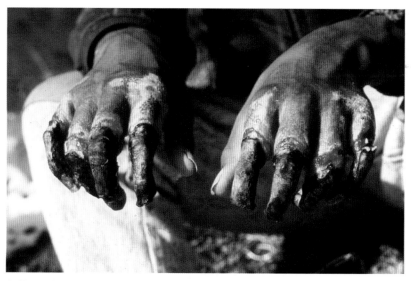

2 Frostbite. Hands of a Tibetan refugee showing a line of demarcation between necrotic (black) and viable tissue four weeks after freezing injury. (L Cook)

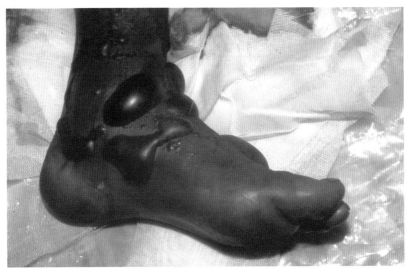

3 Superficial frostbite of a climber's ankle showing blister formation. Complete healing occurred. The cold injury was associated with a fracture of the ankle caused by a fall. (D Murdoch)

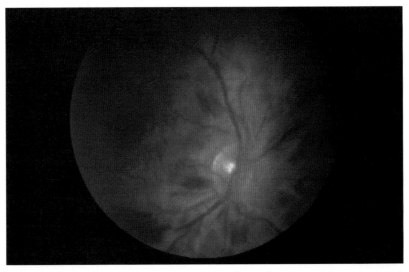

4 Retinal photograph at 5300 m of a climber who later reached the summit of Everest showing vascular engorgement, tortuosity and retinal haemorrhage. (D Depla)

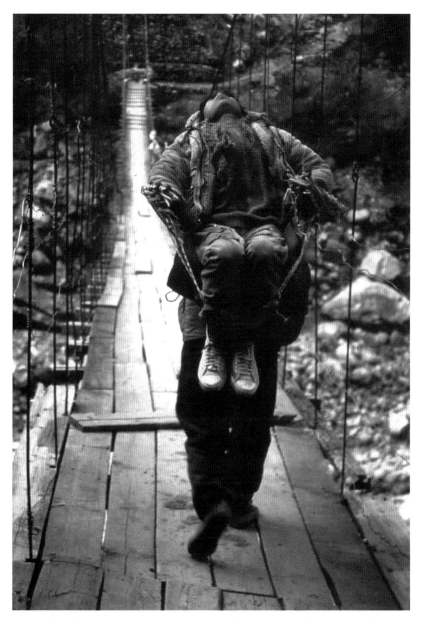
5 A sick climber with high altitude cerebral oedema being carried by a sherpa. (L Cook)

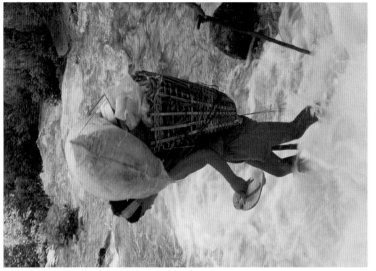

7 River crossing. (A Pollard)

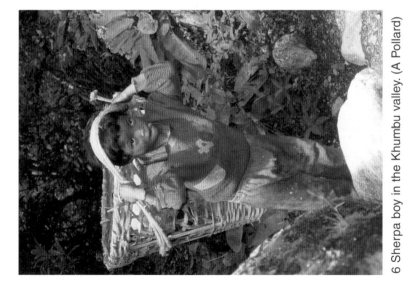

6 Sherpa boy in the Khumbu valley. (A Pollard)

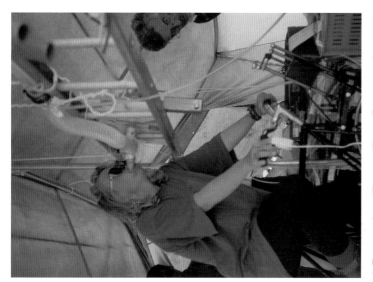

9 Research at Everest Base Camp on the 1994 British Mount Everest Medical Expedition. (A Pollard)

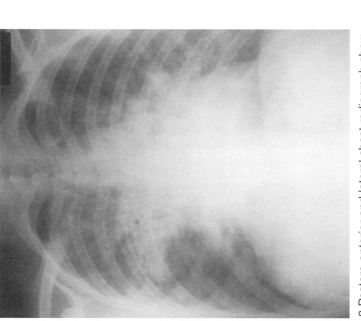

8 Postero-anterior and lateral chest radiograph showing typical appearance of HAPE. (R Price)

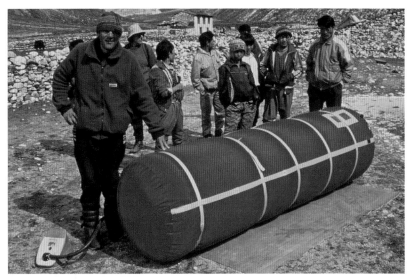

10 The Gamow portable hyperbaric tent. Note this is larger than the more commonly used 'one-person' chamber. (D Murdoch)

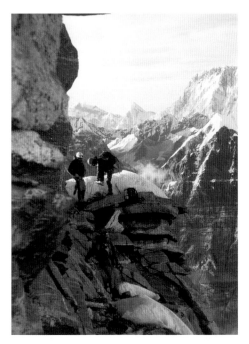

11 Climbers on Chamlang (7319 m) on the first British ascent in 1991. (A Pollard)

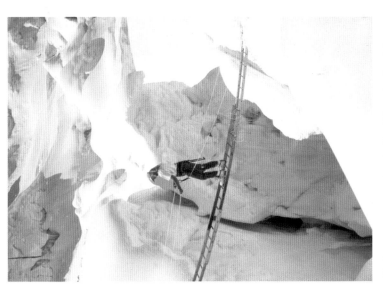

13 Crevasse crossing in the Khumbu icefall, Nepal. (A Pollard)

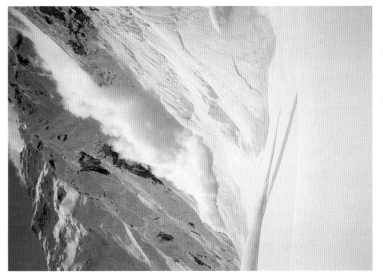

12 Avalanche in the Western Cwm. (A Pollard)

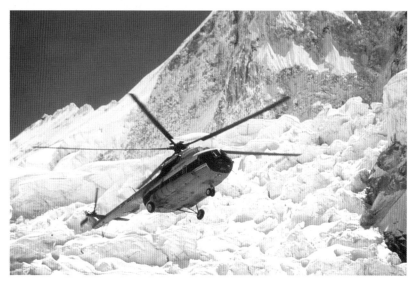

14 Russian Mikoyan-17 helicopter taking off from Everest Base Camp (5300 m) during rescue of a climber suffering from frostbite in 1994. The Khumbu icefall is in the background. (D Collier)

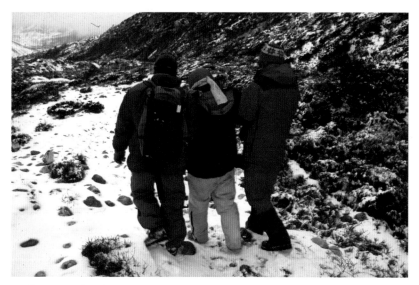

15 Rescue of a climber suffering from damaged ribs. (D Murdoch)

neurological disturbance is the clinical hallmark of heat stroke. Progression to coma and death will occur without treatment. Body temperature must be lowered quickly. In the mountain environment, shielding from the sun and surface cooling (trunk and neck are the most effective areas) with water, snow or even ice should be undertaken urgently. Where evacuation is possible it is still important to commence cooling immediately. Surface cooling is usually continued in hospital, but some advocate peritoneal lavage with cool fluids or mechanical ventilation with cooled humidified air.

Ultraviolet radiation

At high altitude there is an increased risk of exposure to the harmful effects of ultraviolet (UV) radiation from the sun. This is because there is less atmosphere to deflect and absorb the solar radiation, and in addition there is often snow on the ground and surrounding hillsides that reflects the rays and increases the chance of burning, skin ageing and neoplasia. UV light consists of UVA, UVB and UVC. UVC is filtered by the ozone layer. UVB is filtered by the atmosphere more than UVA, but UVB is more damaging to the skin.

Sunscreens should be recommended for climbers and trekkers alike (sun-protection factor (SPF) 15 or greater) and applied to all exposed areas. Lip sunscreens of SPF 15 or greater are necessary to protect the lips. Sunscreens which provide UVA + UVB sunblock with SPF 25 will provide the best protection. Allergic dermatitis may be a problem for some individuals with some sunscreens, and should prompt the use of hypoallergenic preparations such as a high-factor sunscreen for use on children's skin.

Special caution is required if the individual is using drugs which increase photosensitivity.

Box 5.4: Sunburn

- Avoid by using barriers (clothing and sunblock).

Snowblindness

In snowscapes, reflected sun can be very intense. This can result in snow-blindness up to four hours after exposure if appropriate sunglasses with an ultraviolet filter are not worn. Snowblindness usually resolves within 48 hours of onset. Snowblindness is solar damage (sunburn) to the cornea and conjunctiva. It results in a gritty, painful eye with an oedematous eyelid and cornea (best seen with a slit lamp), together with conjunctival oedema and hyperaemia, and it may not appear until the following day. The pain is intense. Topical anaesthetic can be used to examine the eye, but should be avoided thereafter because it is toxic to the corneal epithelium and will reduce awareness of further trauma. However, where descent is necessary over difficult terrain, topical anaesthetics may be required. Treatment consists of oral analgesia (non-steroidal anti-inflammatory drugs should be tried first), topical lubricant (e.g. 1% chloramphenicol), eye pads and a cycloplegic (1% cyclopentolate).

If sunglasses or goggles are lost or broken, and a spare pair is not being carried, snowblindness may be prevented by reducing the amount of light reaching the eye. This can be achieved by cutting small cross-shaped holes to look through, in any material which can be tied around the head over the eyes (e.g. sleeping mat, headband, etc.).

Box 5.5: Snowblindness

- Avoid by using goggles or glasses with a UV filter.
- Always carry a spare pair of glasses/goggles.
- Treat with analgesia, lubrication and cycloplegia.

Chronic exposure of the eye to UV light without adequate UV-filtering sunglasses leads to cataract formation.

References and further reading

Cold injury

Burr RE (1993) Trench foot. *J Wilderness Med.* **4**: 348–52.

Cauchy E, Marsigny B, Allamel G *et al.* (2000) The value of technetium scintigraphy in the prognosis of amputation in severe frostbite injuries of the extremities: a retrospective study of 92 severe frostbite injuries. *J Hand Surg.* **25A**: 969–78.

Cauchy E, Chetaille E, Marchand V *et al.* (2001) Retrospective study of 70 cases of severe frostbite lesions: a proposed new classification scheme. *Wild Environ Med.* **12**: 248–55.

Danzl DF and Pozos RS (1994) Accidental hypothermia. *NEJM.* **331**: 1756–60.

Durrer B and Brugger H (1997) Dilemmas of the rescue doctor in treating hypothermia and frostbite. In: *International Congress of Mountain Medicine Abstract Book.* Interlaken, Switzerland, pp. 42–4.

Durrer B, Brugger H and Syme D (2003) The medical on-site treatment of hypothermia. ICAR–MEDCOM recommendation. *High Alt Med Biol.* **4**: 99–103.

Handley AJ, Golden FStC, Keatinge WR *et al.* (1993) Out-of-hospital management of hypothermia. *J Br Assoc Immed Care.* **16**: 34–5.

Hashmi MA, Bokhari SAH, Rashid M *et al.* (1998) Frostbite: epidemiology at high altitude in the Karakoram mountains. *Ann R Coll Surg Engl.* **80**: 91–5.

Hodkin P, Lowis I, West N *et al.* (1994) *Hypothermia: Report for LDSAMRA Medical Subcommittee.* Lake District Search and Mountain Rescue Association, Keswick.

Lloyd EL (1986) *Hypothermia and Cold Stress.* Croom Helm, London.

Lloyd EL (1994) Temperature and performance. I. Cold. *BMJ.* **309**: 531–4.

Lonning PE, Skulberg A and Abyholm F (1986) Accidental hypothermia. Review of the literature. *Acta Anaesthesiol Scand.* **30**: 601–3.

Murphy JV, Banwell PE, Roberts AHN *et al.* (2000) Frostbite: pathogenesis and treatment. *J Trauma.* **48**: 171–8.

Price RD and Murdoch DR (2001) Perniosis (chilblains) of the thigh: report of five cases, including four following river crossings. *High Alt Med Biol.* **2**: 535–8.

Resuscitation Council (UK) (1996) Cardiac arrest in special circumstances. In: AJ Handley and A Swain (eds) *Advanced Life Support Manual.* Resuscitation Council (UK), London.

Rintamaki H (2000) Predisposing factors and prevention of frostbite. *Int J Circumpol Health.* **59**: 114–21.

Snadden D (1993) The field management of hypothermic casualties arising from Scottish mountain accidents. *Scott Med J.* **38**: 99–103.

Syme D (2002) Position paper: on-site treatment of frostbite for mountaineers. *High Alt Med Biol.* **3**: 297–8.

Tom PA, Garmel GM and Auerbach PS (1994) Environmental-dependent sports emergencies. *Med Clin North Am.* **78**: 305–25.

Weinberg AD (1993) Hypothermia. *Ann Emerg Med.* **22**: 370–7.

Wilson O and Goldman R (1970) Role of air temperature and wind in the time necessary for a finger to freeze. *J Appl Physiol.* **29**: 658–64.

Union Internationale d'Association des Alpinisme (UIAA) Mountain Medical Data Centre Information Sheets, available from the British Mountaineering Council (BMC) Information Service, 177–9 Burton Road, Manchester M20 2BB, UK.

Avalanche

Brugger H and Durrer B (2002) On-site treatment of avalanche victims. ICAR–MEDCOM recommendations. *High Alt Med Biol.* **3**: 421–5.

Brugger H, Durrer B and Adler-Kastner L (1996) On-site triage of avalanche victims with asystole by the emergency doctor. *Resuscitation.* **31**: 11–16.

Brugger H, Durrer B, Adler-Kastner L *et al.* (2001) Field management of avalanche victims. *Resuscitation.* **51**: 7–15.

Falk M, Brugger H and Adler-Kastner L (1994) Avalanche survival chances. *Nature.* **368**: 21.

Heat injury

Clarke CRA and Clark ML (2002) Environmental medicine. In: PJ Kumar and ML Clark (eds) *Clinical Medicine*. Saunders, London, pp. 756–63.

Tek D and Olshaker JS (1992) Heat illness. *Emerg Med Clin North Am*. **10**: 299–310.

Chronic disease, pregnˌ and contraception at altitude

Fitness for altitude

Climbers and trekkers embarking on a trip to high altitude have varied levels of fitness prior to departure. Some will have been training for months before their trip; others will not have taken any regular exercise. At sea level, exercise will improve fitness and prepare the individual for exercise at altitude. All trekkers and climbers should be encouraged to take regular exercise prior to their trip. Sea-level fitness training will not, however, confer protection against altitude illness. Acclimatization is the key to improving performance at altitude.

Asthma

Interestingly, asthma often improves at altitude because the less dense air reduces resistance in the airways (true peak flow measured with a spirometer increases) and there are fewer allergens. Peak flow measurements made with the Mini-Wright peak flow meter are misleading at altitude, as this device is affected by the decrease in air density and under-reads (by 30% at 5300 m) (Pollard *et al.*, 1996). The Mini-Wright measurements may be corrected by adding 6.6% for every 100 mmHg fall in barometric pressure. Trekkers and climbers with asthma should be advised to continue taking their normal sea-level medication, even if symptoms seem to improve. It is unclear what effect lower barometric pressure has on aerosol metered-dose inhalers. Cold air at altitude may precipitate bronchospasm in susceptible individuals. In a group of Swedish

ss-country skiers, repeated exposure to cold air seems to have led to
he development of asthma (Larsson *et al.*, 1993). There is no evidence that
asthmatics are at a greater risk of altitude illness than non-asthmatics.
When an asthmatic becomes breathless at high altitude the possibility of
a diagnosis of HAPE must always be considered although rates of HAPE
are not thought to be higher in this group than in the general population.

Chronic obstructive and interstitial lung disease

With increasing altitude the barometric pressure falls and the partial
pressure of oxygen decreases. Consequently, individuals with respiratory
insufficiency will become increasingly hypoxic. Exercise tolerance will be
reduced and symptoms such as dyspnoea will worsen. Although it may
be advisable for these patients to avoid further hypoxic stress at altitude,
some will still want to take the risk. If ascent is to occur, a slow and cautious
ascent is recommended while continuing to take their usual medication.
A destination should be chosen that allows those with chronic lung
disease to opt out of the higher altitude parts of the trek.

Obstructive sleep apnoea

Individuals with obstructive sleep apnoea who experience arterial oxygen
desaturation during sleep at sea level may find their condition significantly worsens at high altitude. Those residing long term at altitude are at
risk of polycythaemia and possibly chronic mountain sickness.

Sickle-cell disease

Individuals with sickle-cell disease (Hb SS or Hb SC) or trait (Hb AS) have
a high risk of sickle crises at altitudes over 2000 m. Altitude travel should
be avoided. Sickle-cell trait may not be recognized prior to ascent, but
exposure to altitude may precipitate sickling. Treatment of sickling at
altitude is the same as that at sea level (i.e. oxygen, fluids and analgesia).
Descent is a vital component of management.

Coronary artery disease

Individuals with stable coronary artery disease (CAD) tolerate moderate to high altitude exposure relatively well, even while exercising. Indeed, the mortality due to CAD is not increased among residents at intermediate altitudes. However, ascent to these altitudes has precipitated the new onset of angina and an increased severity of angina in those with CAD. Heart failure managed with drug therapy may also decompensate. The greatest risk occurs during the first three days at altitude, and appears to be mainly due to an increase in cardiac work (an initial increase in heart rate and cardiac output) secondary to hypoxia, rather than lack of oxygen to the myocardium itself.

Information is lacking about the risks to those with CAD who ascend to altitudes above 5000 m, although there are plenty of anecdotal examples of individuals with stable CAD performing well at these altitudes. Many recommendations emphasize caution, but in the end it is a personal decision whether to expose oneself to these altitudes or not. However, when making this decision, it is also important to consider the dangers to which rescuers may be exposed should evacuation be necessary.

Individuals with cardiovascular disease need to be counselled about the risk of exposure to environmental hypoxia. If exertional angina is experienced at sea level, it is likely that ascent to high altitude will increase symptoms. Those with well-controlled disease who enjoy a good exercise tolerance at low altitude should manage a high altitude journey, albeit at some added risk. A slow ascent schedule with additional acclimatization days at around 2000 m may be helpful. Immediate descent should occur if symptoms worsen. Recent myocardial infarction and poorly controlled heart failure are contraindications to ascent to high altitude.

There is no evidence that CAD increases susceptibility to or severity of altitude illness.

Hypertension

There are conflicting results from studies of the effects on blood pressure of ascent to high altitude. Changes in blood pressure are probably of a minor degree in both normotensive and hypertensive subjects. There is little evidence that hypertension is associated with adverse events at altitude. Well-controlled hypertension is certainly not a contraindication to travel to high altitude. Doses of antihypertensive agents which are well tolerated at sea level should be continued during altitude travel.

Congenital heart disease

Congenital heart disease occurs in just under 1% of live births. Individuals with congenital cardiac conditions associated with pulmonary hypertension may experience a rise in pulmonary artery pressure, even at moderate altitudes. Although some will tolerate altitude exposure with few adverse circulatory effects, others experience worsening symptoms due to right heart failure. Whether the risks of high altitude exposure are reasonable or not depends on several factors, including the specific condition, whether corrective surgery has been undertaken, and baseline cardiac pressures. A low level of physical activity at altitude should be mandatory.

Diabetes mellitus

A well-controlled diabetic should not experience any adverse event at altitude. However, if there is an increase in energy expenditure above sea-level activity (as is likely on treks or expeditions), then carbohydrate and insulin requirements may alter. In many parts of the world there is a major risk of intercurrent illness (e.g. diarrhoea) precipitating loss of diabetic control. Close attention to blood sugar monitoring is essential, although this may be complicated by inaccurate and inconsistent performance of blood glucose meters above 2000 m (Gautier *et al.*, 1996; Pecchio *et al.*, 2000). Rapidly acting insulins together with regular blood glucose monitoring are preferred because of the potential variation in day-to-day requirements. Glucose should be readily accessible, and companions need to be able to recognize hypoglycaemia and administer sugar or glucagon as appropriate. Hypoglycaemia should be preventable and treatable even in remote wildernesses if diabetics and their companions are well prepared.

Several trekkers have died of diabetic ketoacidosis at high altitude in Nepal in recent years. The possibility that altitude was a risk factor in these cases has been raised, although loss of diabetic control because of intercurrent illness may have been involved.

Useful information from a group of diabetic mountaineers can be found at www.idea2000.org.

Epilepsy

Seizures have been associated with HACE, and there have also been occasional reports of seizures occurring for the first time at high altitude without obvious cause. Epilepsy is not in itself a contraindication to altitude travel. However, a prolonged seizure in a remote setting could be life-threatening, and a seizure occurring on difficult or steep terrain could put the lives of others at risk. If altitude travel is contemplated by an individual with epilepsy, their companions should be familiar with the management of a seizure. Some reassurance may be given by training a companion in the use of rectal diazepam.

Anaemia

There is evidence that a haemoglobin concentration of between 14 and 18 g/dl is optimal for high altitude acclimatization.

Contraception at altitude

Polycythaemia occurs as a response to hypoxia at altitude. The increased blood viscosity resulting from the raised haematocrit may increase the risk of thrombosis associated with oestrogen and some progesterone-containing oral contraceptives. Although many women have used combined oral contraceptives at high altitude with no reported problems, the many examples of stroke and other thrombotic complications at high altitude (*see* page 38) should urge caution for all. Women with other risk factors for thrombosis (history of thrombosis, smoking, family history, etc.) should not use the combined oral contraceptive at altitude (or at sea level). Healthy women with no known risk factors should probably also avoid taking the combined oral contraceptive if they intend to spend more than a week above 4500 m, and should be advised about alternative methods of contraception. Women who are trekking to high altitude for shorter periods (or not going above 4500 m on their trek) should be fully informed about the probable but unquantifiable increased risk of thrombosis and advised about alternative methods of contraception, so that they can make their own decision. There are no specific data on which to base such recommendations, which are therefore based on an assessment of the risk.

Contraceptives can be useful for reducing menstrual loss, which would be convenient on a trek or expedition, although breakthrough bleeding is a problem for some women (Sinclair *et al.*, 1996). Poor absorption of oral contraceptives as a result of gastroenteritis could cause additional problems with breakthrough bleeding. Long periods of physical activity and psychological stress at high altitude can also cause menstrual disturbances and may actually reduce menstrual loss (reviewed by Sinclair *et al.*, 1996). The increased risk of thrombosis at high altitude should always be considered before choosing an oestrogen-containing contraceptive with the intention of reducing menstrual loss. Any change (perhaps to a progesterone-only preparation or depot injection) should be made more than three months before the trip to high altitude in order to reduce the likelihood of menstrual irregularities and other unwanted side-effects. Some sanitary protection should be carried because of the possibility of unexpected menstrual disturbance or withdrawal bleeding as a result of diarrhoea or loss of pills.

Pregnancy and fertility at altitude

Pregnancy at high altitude is associated with intrauterine growth retardation and higher rates of pregnancy-induced hypertension and neonatal hyperbilirubinaemia (Moore, 1987). Those ethnic groups who have been living at high altitude for many generations (e.g. Tibetans) appear to have some protection from these complications, whereas Caucasians are probably the most affected group thus far studied (Zamudio *et al.*, 1993). Current data suggest that high altitude sojourns by unacclimatized pregnant women are best avoided, although brief sojourns to high altitude probably present a relatively small risk. Fertility is reduced in men at altitude as a result of hypoxia to the testes, but returns to normal by two to three weeks after return to sea level.

References and further reading

Fitness for altitude

Levine BD and Stray-Gundersen J (1992) A practical approach to altitude training: where to live and train for optimal performance enhancement. *Int J Sports Med.* **13(Suppl. 1)**: S209–12.

Shlim DR and Gallie J (1992) The causes of death among trekkers in Nepal. *Int J Sports Med.* **13(Suppl. 1)**: S74–6.

Lung disease

Carswell F (1993) Asthma and altitude. *Clin Exp Allergy.* **23**: 973–5.

Larsson K, Ohlsen P, Larsson L *et al.* (1993) High prevalence of asthma in cross-country skiers. *BMJ.* **307**: 1326–9.

Moore LG, Rohr AL, Maisenbach JK *et al.* (1982) Emphysema mortality is increased in Colorado residents at high altitude. *Am Rev Respir Dis.* **126**: 225–8.

Oades PJ, Buchdahl RM and Bush A (1994) Prediction of hypoxaemia at high altitude in children with cystic fibrosis. *BMJ.* **308**: 15–18.

Pollard AJ, Mason NP, Barry PW *et al.* (1996) Effect of altitude on spirometry and the performance of peak flow meters. *Thorax.* **51**: 175–8.

Sue-Chu M, Larsson L and Bjermer L (1996) Prevalence of asthma in young cross-country skiers in central Scandinavia: differences between Norway and Sweden. *Respir Med.* **90**: 99–105.

Heart disease

Alexander JK (1994) Coronary heart disease at altitude. *Tex Heart Inst J.* **21**: 261–6.

Hultgren HN (1992) Effects of altitude upon cardiovascular diseases. *J Wilderness Med*. **3**: 301–8.

Rennie D (1989) Will mountains trekkers have heart attacks? *JAMA*. **261**: 1045–6.

Diabetes

Gautier J-F, Duvallet A, Bigard AX *et al*. (1996) Influence of simulated altitude on the performance of five blood glucose meters. *Diabetes Care*. **19**: 1430–3.

Moore K, Vizzard N, Coleman C *et al*. (2001) Extreme altitude mountaineering and type 1 diabetes: the Diabetes Federation of Ireland Kilimanjaro Expedition. *Diabet Med*. **18**: 749–55.

Pecchio O, Maule S, Migliardi M *et al*. (2000) Effects of exposure at an altitude of 3000 m on performance of glucose meters. *Diabetes Care*. **23**: 129–31.

Contraception

Sinclair J, Cohen J and Hinton E (1996) Use of the oral contraceptive pill on treks and expeditions. *Br J Fam Plann*. **22**: 123–6.

Pregnancy

Moore LG (1987) Altitude-aggravated illness: examples from pregnancy and prenatal life. *Ann Emerg Med*. **16**: 965–73.

Zamudio S, Droma T, Norkyel KY *et al*. (1993) Protection from intrauterine growth retardation in Tibetans at high altitude. *Am J Phys Anthropol*. **91**: 215–24.

7

Training, nutrition and skiing at altitude

Training at altitude for sea-level performance

'Altitude training' refers to exercise training at intermediate altitudes of around 2000 m rather than higher altitudes. Acclimatization at altitude improves the oxygen-carrying capacity of the blood and aids exercise performance. It is nearly impossible to train at the same intensity as that engaged in at sea level when at altitudes above 2300 m, and this reduction in training intensity at altitude (especially over 3000 m) may be of such a magnitude that peak condition cannot be maintained for sea-level competition (Levine and Stray-Gundersen, 1997).

For performance during competition at intermediate altitude, it is preferable to train at the altitude of competition, particularly for endurance events. On the other hand, for athletes competing at sea level, two different regimes of altitude training have been proposed to improve performance, namely living at altitude and training at sea level, or training at altitude (or simulated altitude) and living at sea level.

Living at altitude and training at sea level may offer the greatest physiological advantage for sea-level competition, since the physiological adaptations (especially the increase in red cell mass) favour improved performance, and at the same time training intensity can be maintained because it is undertaken in normoxia (Bailey and Davies, 1997). This training regime seems to provide an advantage for both elite and non-elite athletes (Stray-Gundersen et al., 2001). However, this 'live high, train low' regime only appears to provide an advantage for some individuals, not for all (Chapman et al., 1998). Responders may be individuals who show a more rapid and greater increase in red cell mass during the programme.

Training at altitude may improve oxygen delivery and transfer to skeletal muscle, thereby improving sea-level performance, and this mode of training has been widely used by athletes. However, there are few data to support this approach, and controlled trials have failed to demonstrate a significant advantage. The controversies over altitude training have been reviewed by Hoppeler and Vogt (2001) and Levine and Stray-Gundersen (2001).

Nutrition at altitude

Appetite is reduced at altitude. With acclimatization, appetite returns, but usually remains depressed above 5000 m. Above this height there is evidence for both carbohydrate and fat malabsorption (Dinmore *et al.*, 1994). Fat is frequently unpalatable at these altitudes, and most climbers increase their intake of carbohydrate to compensate for their energy requirements. An average 15% of body weight is lost after three months at 5300–8000 m (Kayser, 1994b).

There is a wide range of views regarding appropriate nutrition at altitude. Certainly on treks and expeditions food is often a major concern for the members of the group, and is memorable after the event. Attention to palatability will improve consumption and enjoyment, particularly at very high altitude where sense of taste seems to be dulled. Iron intake may need to be increased at altitude, particularly in women, to meet the increased demand from the rise in haemoglobin.

Skiing

Altitude illness

Skiing is a popular leisure activity with an international participation of millions. Skiers are exposed to significant altitude in some resorts where reports of altitude illness are not uncommon (Hultgren *et al.*, 1996). Recreational skiers usually ascend rapidly by cable-car or ski-lift, which might increase the likelihood of AMS, but exposure is usually brief before descent. The hotel and *après-ski* are usually located in the valley at a relatively safe low elevation. Symptoms of AMS may be mistakenly attributed to alcohol ingestion or unaccustomed exercise. High resorts with sleeping altitudes above 2500 m are particularly likely to precipitate altitude illness in skiers who ascend rapidly. Ski-mountaineers usually have higher sleeping sites (e.g. Alpine huts) than downhill skiers, and mild AMS is common. HAPE and HACE may also occur. Most skiing occurs in resorts where rescue is rapid except in bad weather, and altitude illness can be readily treated by rapid descent.

Ski sickness

Ski sickness, a form of motion sickness, occurs in susceptible individuals (notably those with myopia or astigmatism) in conditions of poor visibility when visual, vestibular and peripheral sensory information is conflicting (Hausler, 1995). Symptoms include dizziness with rotatory or pendular sensations, nausea and vomiting. In severe cases, vestibular sedatives (hyoscine, cinnarizine) or antihistamines could be considered.

Cardiovascular fitness and skiing

Many skiers normally have a sedentary lifestyle and their annual skiing trip may produce unaccustomed cardiovascular stress. Skiers should be encouraged to maintain fitness throughout the year. Silent ischaemic episodes are common in individuals who ski who have previously had a myocardial infarct (Volker *et al.*, 1990). The incidence and duration of ischaemia are reduced by nitrate prophylaxis.

Injuries

Injuries occur in up to five per 1000 downhill skiers and snowboarders through collision with fellow skiers or trees or other inanimate objects (Bladin and McCrory, 1995; Davidson and Laliotis, 1996a). Injuries in cross-country skiers tend to be of a more minor nature and occur at a rate of 0.5 per 1000 skier days (Renstrom and Johnson, 1989). Other injuries result during falls when ski-bindings fail to separate. Most notable injuries include soft tissue injuries, fractures and more severe abdominal, spinal (skiing accounts for 5% of all spinal injuries in Canada), head and chest trauma (Reid and Saboe, 1989). On New Zealand skifields, the most common injuries involve the face and hands. With modern ski-bindings, lower leg fractures are relatively rare.

Snowboarders are as likely to injure their wrists or ankles as their knees, while knee injuries are the most common injury in skiing, accounting for about 35% of all injuries (Davidson and Laliotis, 1996a, 1996b). They usually involve damage to the medial collateral ligament. Skier's knee is a triad of torn medial collateral ligament, ruptured medial meniscus and rupture of the anterior cruciate ligament. All other knee ligaments may be injured. Initial management requires immobilization of the knee and provision of pain relief. Specialist advice will be required for further management (Paletta and Warren, 1994; Steadman and Sterett, 1995). Control of effusion with rest, ice and elevation should commence immediately. Drainage of the effusion should be avoided if sterility cannot be guaranteed, but may occasionally be required to facilitate evacuation.

Skier's or gamekeeper's thumb is used to describe a tear of the ulnar collateral ligament of the thumb metacarpophalangeal joint, caused by a fall while the ski pole is still held in the hand, forcing the thumb radially (Fricker and Hintermann, 1995). Surgery is often required.

In general, the management of skiing injuries depends on the situation. First-aid measures may be all that are needed if helicopter rescue is readily available. When an injury occurs a long way from medical support, the approach will be directed towards stabilization and safe evacuation, which is discussed in detail in Chapter 9.

Many skiing injuries may be avoided by careful preparation (fitness conditioning, especially for sedentary individuals, focusing on the legs and back), use of appropriate equipment (for age, size and expertise) that has been correctly adjusted, skiing under control at speeds that are consistent with ability, and resting before fatigue becomes the limiting factor (Hunter, 1999). Many skiing injuries involve alcohol consumption and most occur on prepared slopes (the piste). Objective danger from avalanche, crevasses and lightning strike is more likely to affect ski-mountaineers off-piste.

Various devices are available to help with finding individuals buried in an avalanche (avalanche transceivers/Pieps). The world standard frequency for avalanche transceivers is 457 kHz. These devices should be carried by all members of a party who ski off-piste in order to enable companions and rescuers to find casualties. Appropriate travel and health insurance should be obtained with cover extended to include winter sports and helicopter rescue.

Preparation for ski-mountaineering should involve training in recognizing safe snow conditions, avoiding avalanche-prone slopes and crevasse rescue.

References and further reading

Training at high altitude for sea-level performance

Bailey DM and Davies B (1997) Physiological implications of altitude training for endurance performance at sea level: a review. *Br J Sports Med.* **31**: 183–90.

Chapman RF, Stray-Gundersen J and Levine BD (1998) Individual variation in response to altitude training. *J Appl Physiol.* **85**: 1448–56.

Hoppeler H and Vogt M (2001) Hypoxia training for sea-level performance. In: RC Roach, PD Wagner and PH Hackett (eds) *Hypoxia: from genes to the bedside*. Kluwer Academic, New York, pp. 61–73.

Levine BD (2002) Intermittent hypoxic training: fact and fancy. *High Alt Med Biol.* **3**: 177–93.

Levine BD and Stray-Gundersen J (1997) 'Living high – training low': effect of moderate-altitude acclimatization with low-altitude training on performance. *J Appl Physiol.* **83**: 102–12.

Levine BD and Stray-Gundersen J (2001) The effects of altitude training are mediated primarily by acclimatization, rather than by hypoxic exercise. In: RC Roach, PD Wagner and PH Hackett (eds) *Hypoxia: from genes to the bedside*. Kluwer Academic, New York, pp. 75–88.

Levine BD, Roach RC and Houston CS (1992) Work and training at altitude. In: JR Sutton, G Coates and CS Houston (eds) *Hypoxia and Mountain Medicine*. Queen City Printers, Burlington, VT.

Stray-Gundersen J, Chapman RF and Levine BD (2001) 'Living high – training low': altitude training improves sea-level performance in male and female elite runners. *J Appl Physiol.* **91**: 1113–20.

Nutrition at altitude

Dinmore AJ, Edwards JSA, Menzies IS *et al*. (1994) Intestinal carbohydrate absorption and permeability at high altitude (5730 m). *J Appl Physiol*. **76**: 1903–7.

Kayser B (1994a) *Factors limiting exercise performance in man at high altitude* (PhD thesis). Geneva University, Geneva.

Kayser B (1994b) Nutrition and energetics of exercise at altitude. *Sports Med*. **17**: 309–23.

Westerterp KR (2001) Energy and water balance at high altitude. *News Physiol Sci*. **16**: 134–7.

Skiing

Bladin C and McCrory P (1995) Snowboarding injuries. An overview. *Sports Med*. **19**: 358–64.

Davidson TM and Laliotis AT (1996a) Alpine skiing injuries: a nine-year study. *West J Med*. **164**: 310–14.

Davidson TM and Laliotis AT (1996b) Snowboarding injuries: a four-year study with comparison with alpine ski injuries. *West J Med*. **164**: 231–7.

Fricker R and Hintermann B (1995) Skier's thumb. Treatment, prevention and recommendations. *Sports Med*. **19**: 73–9.

Hausler R (1995) Ski sickness. *Acta Otolaryngol (Stockh)*. **115**: 1–2.

Hultgren HN, Honigman B, Theis K *et al*. (1996) High-altitude pulmonary edema at a ski resort. *West J Med*. **164**: 222–7.

Hunter RE (1999) Skiing injuries. *Am J Sports Med*. **27**: 381–9.

Paletta GA and Warren RF (1994) Knee injuries and alpine skiing. Treatment and rehabilitation. *Sports Med*. **17**: 411–23.

Reid DC and Saboe L (1989) Spine fractures in winter sports. *Sports Med*. **7**: 393–9.

Renstrom P and Johnson RJ (1989) Cross-country skiing injuries and biomechanics. *Sports Med.* **8**: 346–70.

Steadman JR and Sterett WI (1995) The surgical treatment of knee injuries in skiers. *Med Sci Sports Exerc.* **27**: 328–33.

Volker K, Hoppe B, Krestin M *et al.* (1990) Cross-country and downhill skiing in patients with myocardial infarct. Can silent ischaemia be prevented by drug therapy? *Fortschr Med.* **108**: 273–5.

8

Travel related diseases and vaccination

Malaria

Malaria transmission does not occur at altitudes above 2000–2500 m, and in some parts of the world the ceiling is lower. In Nepal, for example, there is a very low risk of acquiring malaria above 1300 m. However, travellers often pass through malarious areas on their way to or from high altitude destinations. As most prophylactic antimalarial drugs should be taken for four weeks after leaving a malarious area, many trekkers and climbers will need to take antimalarials while in the high mountains. Table 8.1 highlights some malarious areas near popular high altitude destinations. Recent publications and current advice from local travel medicine authorities should be consulted for information on the recommended antimalarial regimens for specific regions, although it should be noted that chloroquine resistance has been reported in almost all of the regions mentioned in Table 8.1.

Of the antimalarials, mefloquine may be best avoided in mountaineers because this drug may cause vertigo and dizziness, and is thus contraindicated for those whose activities require fine co-ordination and spatial discrimination. The newer antimalarial, Malarone, has the advantage of a regimen that finishes only one week after leaving a malarious area (compared with four weeks for other prophylactic antimalarials).

Standby therapy (also known as emergency self-treatment) is an alternative to continuous antimalarial prophylaxis, and is especially suited to travellers whose exposure to malarious areas is brief and/or intermittent. Travellers carry treatment courses of antimalarials for use in situations in which malaria is suspected and medical assistance is not available.

Table 8.1: Some malarious areas near popular high altitude destinations

Country	Malarious areas
Afghanistan	Below 2000 m (May to November)
Bhutan	Southern belt of Chirang, Samchi, Samdrupjongkhar, Sarpang and Shemgang
India	Below 2000 m
Nepal	Rural areas of the Terai districts below 1300 m
New Guinea	Below 1800 m
Pakistan	Below 2000 m
Tajikistan	Especially southern border areas (Khatlon region), in some central (Dunshanbe), western (Gorno-Badakhshan) and northern (Leninabad region) areas (June to October)
Ethiopia	Below 2000 m
Kenya	Little risk in Nairobi and above 2500 m
Tanzania	Below 1800 m
Uganda	Below 2000 m
Bolivia	Below 2500 m in the departments of Beni, Pando, Santa Cruz and Tarija, and in the provinces of Lacareja, Rurenabaque, and North and South Yungas in La Paz Department. Lower risk in Cochabamba and Chuquisaca
Colombia	High risk in rural/jungle areas below 800 m
Ecuador	Below 1500 m
Peru	Below 2500 m
Mexico	High risk in the states of Chiapas, Quintana Roo, Sinaloa and Tabasco, and moderate risk in the states of Chichuahua, Durango, Nayarit, Oaxaca and Sonora

Suitable drugs for this purpose are mefloquine, sulphadoxine-pyrimethamine, quinine and (in areas without chloroquine resistance) chloroquine.

Travellers' diarrhoea

Many high altitude regions of the world are situated in countries where there is a high risk of acute diarrhoeal illness in travellers (20–50%). At least 80% of cases of travellers' diarrhoea have an infectious aetiology. In most cases the pathogen is bacterial, with enterotoxigenic *Escherichia coli* continuing to be the most commonly encountered organism. Viruses, including rotavirus and Norwalk agent, and protozoa such as *Giardia lamblia*, *Entamoeba histolytica*, *Cryptosporidium* and *Cyclospora* are also important causes of travellers' diarrhoea, although their impact may be limited to specific locations and seasons.

In most cases, travellers' diarrhoea is a mild, self-limiting illness lasting two to four days. However, associated nausea, vomiting and abdominal pain may severely disrupt travel plans and create dangerous situations high on a mountain. Furthermore, preliminary evidence suggests that those with diarrhoea have a higher incidence of acute mountain sickness.

Identifying the causative organism by clinical symptoms and signs is difficult, although some features are suggestive. Dysentery (bloody diarrhoea) is usually due to an invasive organism such as *Salmonella*, *Shigella*, *Campylobacter* or *Entamoeba histolytica*. Watery diarrhoea is usually due to enterotoxigenic *E. coli*, *Cryptosporidium* or a viral pathogen, while vomiting is the major symptom with many viral infections. Persistent diarrhoea (duration longer than two weeks) may suggest *Giardia* or *Cyclospora*.

Prevention

Needless to say, avoiding the ingestion of enteropathogens is the best way to prevent travellers' diarrhoea. Untreated water should be avoided (methods of water purification are discussed in Chapter 10). It is also important to avoid undercooked and reheated food, unpeelable fruit and ice cubes. The use of antimicrobial chemoprophylaxis remains controversial. Although the use of these agents has reduced attack rates by as much as 80–90%, there are potential problems. These include the risk of adverse effects (e.g. skin rashes, vaginal candidiasis, photosensitivity reactions), the false sense of security that may be imparted, and the difficulty formulating a treatment plan should diarrhoea occur while on prophylaxis. In addition, widespread use will increase bacterial resistance.

Chemoprophylaxis should not be used if the period of risk exceeds three weeks, because of the increased risk of adverse reactions, and should probably be reserved for certain high-risk groups (travellers with underlying chronic illness which may be exacerbated by gastroenteritis, those who cannot be sure that the food they eat will be safely prepared, cases where illness would jeopardize the trip). The most effective agents for chemoprophylaxis are the quinolones (e.g. ciprofloxacin), cotrimoxazole being less effective for most areas of the world. The potentially serious side-effects of cotrimoxazole (trimethoprim-sulphamethoxazole) have limited its use in the UK. Trimethoprim used alone does not seem to be so effective (60% reduction in attack rate compared with 85% reduction using cotrimoxazole). Widespread resistance has developed to ampicillin and doxycycline. Recommended adult doses are as follows:

Agent	Dosage
Norfloxacin	400 mg daily
Ciprofloxacin	500 mg daily
Cotrimoxazole	160/800 mg daily
Bismuth subsalicylate	Two tablets with meals and at bedtime.

The use of quinolones is difficult to justify for prophylaxis in children because of the risk of cartilage toxicity as seen in animal studies. There have been no trials of other agents, and therefore none can be recommended in children.

Treatment

The treatment of travellers' diarrhoea includes replacement of fluid and electrolyte losses, antimicrobial chemotherapy and the use of antimotility agents. Although food stimulates the gastrocolic reflex, it should not be withheld, and people should be encouraged to eat what they desire. Antimicrobials reduce the duration and severity of disease and may be effective as a single dose. After initiation of treatment, diarrhoea typically lasts about one day, whereas it lasts two to four days if untreated. As with antimicrobial chemoprophylaxis, quinolones are the most effective. Increasing resistance to ampicillin and doxycycline limit the use of these agents. The best results have been achieved with a combination of an antimicrobial agent and the antimotility agent loperamide in adults. It should be noted, however, that antimotility agents are contraindicated in children and when the diarrhoea is bloody (dysentery).

For persisting symptoms when *Giardia* is suspected, commence metronidazole or tinidazole. *Cyclospora* has been implicated as a common cause of prolonged (more than three weeks) diarrhoea in Nepal, and is effectively treated with cotrimoxazole (Hoge *et al.*, 1995).

Adults

One approach to the treatment of travellers' diarrhoea is as follows. For moderate to severe diarrhoea (three loose motions per day), try single-dose antimicrobial therapy plus loperamide. If symptoms are no better after 12 hours, continue with standard dosing for a full three-day course. For severe diarrhoea with incapacitating symptoms or fever or bloody motions, commence an antimicrobial agent at standard doses for three days. Single doses may be insufficient to eradicate salmonella infection. The agents and dosage regimens for the treatment of travellers' diarrhoea are listed in Table 8.2.

Table 8.2: Agents and dosage regimens for the treatment of travellers' diarrhoea

Agent		Dosage
Norfloxacin		800 mg once *or* 400 mg bd for three days
Ciprofloxacin	– adults	1000 mg once *or* 500 mg bd for three days
	– children	5–10 mg/kg per dose bd for three days (maximum 750 mg)
Cotrimoxazole	– adults	320/1600 mg once *or* 160/800 mg bd for three days
	– children	5/25 mg/kg bd for three days
Metronidazole	– adults	2 g daily as a single dose for three days
	– children	7.5 mg/kg/dose tds for three days (maximum 800 mg)
Tinidazole	– adults	2 g daily as a single dose for three days
	– children	50 mg/kg as a single dose for three days
Loperamide	– adults	4 mg initially, then 2 mg after each loose motion (maximum 16 mg/day)

bd = to be taken twice daily; tds = to be taken three times daily.

Children

In children, oral rehydration is the mainstay of treatment. Packets or sachets of commercially available electrolyte mixtures should always be recommended, since home-made recipes are often incorrectly prepared and may lead to hypernatraemia. Although traditional teaching has been to stop solid and milk feeds in infants and children with acute diarrhoea and give oral rehydration solution for 24 hours, this practice can no longer be supported. Oral rehydration is still the priority during acute diarrhoea, but laboratory and clinical data now persuade that breast milk, full-strength bottle milk and age-appropriate solid feeds should also be continued (Duggan and Nurko, 1997). Continuation of feeding does not worsen the diarrhoea, but leads to a nutritional advantage and may decrease stool output and shorten the duration of diarrhoea.

Antimotility agents should be avoided. Antibiotic therapy is helpful, but choice of agent is difficult. Cotrimoxazole is preferred by many, and is recommended in the USA, but potential serious side-effects have reduced enthusiasm in the UK. In a remote setting, antibiotic therapy may reduce the severity and duration of diarrhoea and prevent life-threatening dehydration or septicaemia (young children are more likely to get invasive disease with bacterial enteritis). In this situation, a five-day course of ciprofloxacin can be used. Recent data suggest that single short courses do not cause any joint toxicity and are safe (Bethell *et al.*, 1996).

Jet lag

Jet lag occurs following rapid flight across several time zones to the east or west, and is especially common after time-zone changes of more than 5 hours. It is characterized by fatigue, loss of concentration, and inability to sleep at the new night-time. In general, eastward flights are associated with greater sleep disruption than westward flights. In addition, adjustment to the new time zone tends to be slower after eastward flights (about 1 hour per day after eastward flights and 1.5 hours per day after westward flights).

There are several ways to minimize the effects of jet lag.

Pre-travel counter-measures

1   Add a stopover of at least a day to break up the journey if possible.

2   Obtain a full night's sleep for 2–3 days before departure.

3   Avoid planning important activities immediately after arrival at the new time zone.

Counter-measures during aircraft flight

1   Set your watch to the new time zone on departure, and try to adjust your eating and sleeping times accordingly.

After arrival at destination

1   Try to sleep at the local time.

2   Take naps (of less than 1 hour) during the adjustment time. Naps are important for topping up total sleep time and for improving alertness during the day.

3   Minimize alcohol consumption.

4   Exposure to sunlight or other bright light will aid adjustment.

5   Melatonin.

6   Hypnotics.

The hormone melatonin may have a role both in alleviating the symptoms of jet lag and in promoting adjustment of the body clock. Melatonin clearly relieves fatigue and promotes sleep and alertness at the new time zone after both eastward and westward travel. In general, it is recommended that melatonin is taken around 20.00–22.00 hours local time after arrival at a new destination for 3 to 4 days for both eastward and westward flights. Some authors also recommend a dose at 18.00–19.00 hours local time on the day of departure for eastward flights. Most studies of the use of melatonin to treat jet lag have used doses of 5 mg, although doses of 2–3 mg have also been used. The main side-effect of melatonin is drowsiness. Consequently, activities that involve driving or operating machinery should be avoided for 4–5 hours after administration of the drug.

Benzodiazepines may be useful for promotion of sleep during the first 2 to 3 nights in a new time zone. However, they have not been shown to assist adjustment of the body clock, and they may have residual detrimental effects on alertness and psychomotor performance. In general, benzodiazepines should only be used when other measures are ineffective, and should always be taken at the lowest effective dose. Drugs with shorter half-lives may have fewer residual effects.

Motion sickness

Motion sickness is a frequently debilitating illness that occasionally accompanies passive transportation by sea, air or road. It is characterized by nausea, vomiting, cold sweats, pallor and yawning. The cause of motion sickness is incompletely understood, although disturbed labyrinthine function is involved, probably as a consequence of conflicting inputs to the brain from visual and labyrinthine sensors. Although a variety of changes in speed and direction can cause motion sickness, up-and-down movement is the most powerful inducer. A characteristic feature of motion sickness is the ability to habituate to the causative environmental stimuli. This adaptation is motion specific and may not necessarily transfer to different modes of transportation. For example, passengers who have adapted to travel on a large ship frequently become seasick once they are transferred to a small boat. Adaptation is lost after the stimulus has been discontinued for a few days.

Several measures can be taken to help to prevent or minimize motion sickness. These include the following:

1 restricting visual activity by gazing at the horizon, minimizing fixation on close moving objects, and avoiding reading (if possible, closing the eyes and lying flat can be useful)

2 minimizing body movements

3 ensuring that there is good ventilation

Table 8.3: Prophylaxis of motion sickness

Medication	Dose	Duration of protective effect
Cinnarizine	20 mg	4 hours
Domperidone	15 mg	Second dose after 4 hours
Cyclizine	50 mg	> 4 hours
Dimenhydrinate	50 mg	4 hours
Caffeine	50 mg	
Ginger root	250 mg	4 hours
		Second dose after 4 hours
Meclozine	12.5 mg	12 hours
Caffeine	10 mg	
Cinnarizine	25 mg	> 6 hours
		Second dose the following morning
Scopolamine	0.5 mg transdermal patch	72 hours

Adapted from Schmid *et al.* (1994) *J Travel Med.* **1**: 203–6.

4   avoiding potentially noxious stimuli, large meals and alcohol

5   engaging in distracting activities.

Many drugs have been used in an attempt to prevent motion sickness. Of these, antihistamines and phenothiazines are the most popular. Both of these groups of drugs may cause anticholinergic side-effects, which (especially drowsiness) can be problematic. Table 8.3 lists the details of the most commonly used prophylactic agents.

Rabies

Rabies is an acute, invariably fatal encephalomyelitis that is almost always transmitted through the bite of an infected mammal, especially dogs. The risk of developing rabies is greatest with bites that cause bleeding, are on the head and neck, or are caused by bats. The first symptoms are paraesthesiae, burning and pruritus at the site of the bite as invasion of the nervous system begins. Subsequently the whole limb may become involved, and typically fever and anxiety develop. As the virus spreads to the central nervous system, either encephalitic (furious, 70%) or paralytic (dumb, 30%) rabies may occur. Coma and then death occur within 2 days to 4 weeks after the onset of symptoms. Rabies kills up to 60 000 people every year worldwide. The majority of the reported deaths from rabies occur in Asia, particularly India and Bangladesh. Most of the remaining deaths are reported from the Philippines, Sri Lanka, Thailand, the Americas and Africa. However, rabies is endemic worldwide except in a few countries that have been certified as rabies free by the World Health Organization.

The most important aspect of rabies prevention is the avoidance of potentially infected animals. Pre-exposure prophylaxis is considered in some circumstances for individuals travelling to areas where there is a high level of endemicity, particularly where dogs are the main reservoir of disease.

Local treatment of a rabid wound reduces transmission. Therefore following a bite from a potentially rabid animal, bites and wounds should immediately be thoroughly and vigorously washed with soap and water, detergent or water alone. If available, a virucidal agent (e.g. 70% alcohol or iodine solution) should then be applied to the wound. Suturing of the wound should be delayed for 1 to 2 days if at all possible.

Vaccination is almost completely effective in preventing rabies following exposure if it is undertaken early enough. However, it is reasonable to institute post-exposure prophylaxis even if 6 months have elapsed since the exposure. In previously unimmunized individuals with a significant exposure, human diploid cell vaccine (HDCV) is administered on days 0, 3, 7, 14 and 28 by intramuscular injection into the deltoid region (or the thigh in a small child). Human rabies immunoglobulin (HRIG) should be administered intramuscularly with the first dose of vaccine to provide protection until host immunity develops in response to the vaccine. Half of the HRIG dose should be infiltrated around the wound to neutralize virus in the tissues. A double first dose of vaccine is recommended for multiple severe bites in children. In previously immunized individuals, where there has been clear documentation of complete pre-exposure immunization, HRIG is not required, but two booster doses of HDCV should be administered on day 0 and day 3.

Leptospirosis

Leptospirosis is of greatest risk to travellers who are engaged in activities involving contact with water, such as canoeing, swimming or caving. The disease is endemic in the tropics and other parts of the world, and infection is transmitted through exposure to water or soil contaminated with urine from infected animals. Many animals can serve as reservoirs, and the major carriers vary between different regions. Clinical manifestations include an acute generalized febrile illness, jaundice, renal failure, meningitis and pneumonitis. Prevention involves minimizing contact with potentially contaminated water.

Venomous bites and stings

Bees, wasps and hornets rarely cause serious direct toxicity as a result of their venom. However, anaphylaxis from such stings is a risk in individuals with hypersensitivity. When this condition is recognized, adrenaline (epinephrine) should be carried.

Most snake bites do not involve venom that is dangerous to humans, but some species are capable of injecting sufficient venom to be lethal.

Most such bites occur on the limbs. Treatment consists of reassurance, immobilization of the affected limb, analgesia and immediate hospital medical advice. All other treatments and remedies should be avoided. Antivenom is indicated if there are signs of spontaneous bleeding (mucous membranes, haematuria), neurological signs, cardiovascular compromise, or swelling of more than half of the bitten limb. Unless the species of snake can be identified, a polyvalent venom is used that covers the locally prevalent species. Anaphylaxis is a major risk after antivenom, and adrenaline (epinephrine) should be available. If toxic effects of snake bites do occur, supportive therapy may be necessary to manage haemorrhage, respiratory paralysis, cardiovascular collapse and secondary infection.

Scorpion stings are not usually fatal in adults, but are very painful and can lead to catecholamine release. Dangerous scorpions are found in India, Africa, the Middle East, and North, South and Central America.

Spider bites are unpleasant but are rarely life-threatening in adults. Antivenom for dangerous species is available in some countries. The most dangerous species are the black widow spider, banana spider and funnel-web spider (which can cause cardiovascular compromise and neurological symptoms), and the brown recluse spider (which can cause local necrosis, coagulopathy and haemoglobinuria). Dangerous spiders are found in Australia, South Africa, the Mediterranean countries and North, South and Central America.

Leeches

Leeches are common in warm wet climates, and may be found as high as 3500 m. They are most prevalent in the monsoon and early post-monsoon seasons, and feed on the blood of wild and domestic animals and humans. They are usually acquired from vegetation to which the leech is attached, awaiting a passing animal. The leech attaches to the skin by its mouth-parts and painlessly feeds on blood from superficial vessels using an anticoagulant (hirudin), a histamine-like vasodilator, a local anaesthetic and hyaluronidase.

Some trekkers may find leeches very disturbing, and the psychological effects are usually far in excess of any local skin damage. Bleeding is not usually a problem, but epistaxis, tracheal obstruction and haematemesis have been described when leeches have found their way into respective orifices. The risk of hepatitis B transmission remains uncertain. Several techniques have been used to remove leeches, including flicking, and application of salt or a lighted match. One drop of iodine from the stock carried to treat water is immediately effective in making the leech drop off, and seems to be superior to other methods.

Vaccinations

Vaccinations are recommended for many high altitude destinations. Recommendations vary over time and from source to source. It is therefore important to seek up-to-date information at least six weeks before departure. The following is a general guide to various regions of the world.

Europe, USA, Canada, Japan, Australia, New Zealand and Antarctica

No particular vaccinations are recommended apart from tetanus. Tick-borne encephalitis is a risk to hikers in some of the warm forested areas of central and eastern Europe and Scandinavia. A vaccine is available, but may be difficult to obtain outside Europe. Diphtheria vaccination is recommended for travel to the countries that comprised the former Soviet Union.

Asia

Tetanus, typhoid and hepatitis A vaccines are recommended. Meningococcal (A/C) vaccine is recommended for Nepal, India north of Delhi and Saudi Arabia. Individuals who plan to spend lengthy periods in some rural (especially rice-growing) areas may consider Japanese B encephalitis virus vaccination. Polio vaccine may be recommended for the Indian subcontinent.

Africa

Tetanus, polio, typhoid and hepatitis A vaccines are recommended. Yellow fever vaccination is compulsory, and meningococcal vaccination is recommended for many countries in central, western and eastern Africa.

Central and South America

Tetanus, typhoid and hepatitis A vaccines are recommended for many areas. Yellow fever vaccination is recommended for regions from Panama to the Amazon basin. Meningococcal vaccine should be considered for travel in rural Brazil.

Pacific islands

Tetanus, typhoid and hepatitis A vaccines are recommended for many areas.

Yellow fever is currently the only compulsory vaccination for some countries, and may also be required for certain countries following travel from a country endemic for yellow fever. Travellers to rural areas in Asia, Africa and South America may consider rabies vaccination.

References and further reading

Travellers' diarrhoea

Bethell DB, Hien TT, Phi LT et al. (1996) Effects on growth of single short courses of fluoroquinolones. *Arch Dis Child*. **74**: 44–6.

Duggan C and Nurko S (1997) Feeding the gut: the scientific basis for continued enteral nutrition during acute diarrhoea. *J Pediatr*. **131**: 801–8.

DuPont HL and Ericsson CD (1993) Prevention and treatment of travelers' diarrhea. *NEJM*. **328**: 1821–7.

Farthing MJG (1994) Travellers' diarrhoea. *Gut*. **35**: 1–4.

Gentile DA and Kennedy BC (1991) Wilderness medicine for children. *Pediatrics*. **88**: 967–81.

Hoge CW, Shlim DR, Ghimire M et al. (1995) Placebo-controlled trial of cotrimoxazole for cyclospora infections among travellers and foreign residents in Nepal. *Lancet*. **345**: 691–3.

Meyer K (1994) *How to Shit in the Woods*. Ten Speed Press, Berkeley, CA.

Rendi-Wagner P and Kollaritsch H (2002) Drug prophylaxis for travelers' diarrhea. *Clin Infect Dis*. **34**: 628–33.

Salam I, Katelaris P, Leigh-Smith S *et al*. (1994) Randomised trial of single-dose ciprofloxacin for travellers' diarrhoea. *Lancet.* **344**: 1537–9.

Wilson-Howarth J (2000) *Shitting Pretty*. Travellers' Tales, San Francisco, CA.

Leeches

Kraemer BA, Korber KE, Aquino TI *et al*. (1988) Use of leeches in plastic and reconstructive surgery: a review. *J Reconstr Microsurg.* **2**: 201–3.

Tropical and travel medicine

British National Formulary, British Medical Association and Royal Pharmaceutical Society of Great Britain (2003) *Malaria Prophylaxis*. British National Formulary, British Medical Association and Royal Pharmaceutical Society of Great Britain, London.

Centers for Disease Control (1990) *Health Information for International Travel*. US Department of Health and Human Services, Atlanta, GA.

Commonwealth Department of Health, Housing and Community Services (1991) *Health Information for International Travel* (3e). Australian Government Publishing Service, Canberra.

Cook GC (ed.) (1996) *Manson's Tropical Diseases* (20e). WB Saunders, London.

Davies EG, Elliman DAC, Hart CA *et al*. (1996) *Manual of Childhood Infections*. WB Saunders, Philadelphia, PA.

Dawood R (2002) *Travellers' Health. How to stay healthy abroad*. Oxford University Press, Oxford.

Feigin RD and Cherry JD (1997) *Textbook of Paediatric Infectious Disease* (4e). WB Saunders, Philadelphia, PA.

Department of Health (1992) *Health Advice for Travellers*. HMSO, London.

Department of Health. *Health Information for Overseas Travel*. HMSO, London (published annually).

Department of Health (1996) *Immunisation Against Infectious Disease*. HMSO, London.

Mandell GL, Bennett JE and Dolin R (eds) (2000) *Principles and Practice of Infectious Disease* (5e). Churchill Livingstone, New York.

Patel AC and Ellis-Pegler R (1992) *Health Advice for Overseas Travellers.* Department of Health (New Zealand), Wellington.

Pollard AJ and Murdoch DR (2001) *Fast Facts: travel medicine.* Health Press, Oxford.

Ryan R (1995) *Stay Healthy Abroad.* Health Education Authority, London.

Schmid R, Schick T, Steffen R *et al.* (1994) Comparison of seven commonly used agents for prophylaxis of seasickness. *J Travel Med.* **1**: 203–6.

Walker E, Williams G and Raeside F (1993) *ABC of Healthy Travel* (4e). BMJ Publishing Group, London.

Werner D (1993) *Where There is No Doctor.* Available from TALC (Teaching Aids at Low Cost), PO Box 49, St Albans, Herts AL1 5TX, UK.

World Health Organization. *International Travel and Health: vaccination requirements and health advice.* World Health Organization, Geneva (published annually).

9

Prevention and management of illness and injury on mountains

Mountain skills, communications and mountain rescue

An important aspect of preventative medicine on mountains involves ensuring that a party has the appropriate skills. Novice climbers and ski-mountaineers may suffer accidents or injuries which might be avoidable if either some prior training in basic mountain skills was undertaken or an experienced mountaineer accompanied the party. A comprehensive discussion of rock, snow or ice mountaineering skills and techniques is beyond the scope of this book, but a number of books and courses are available which may be helpful in equipping the novice mountaineer with the necessary ability (*see* Further reading and Appendix 8, Useful addresses).

All members of a party should be familiar with the use of a map and compass, and mountaineers will need to be adequately equipped and proficient in basic rope techniques and the use of safety equipment, including a helmet and harness. Navigation is greatly aided in remote settings by the use of handheld global positioning devices which accurately pinpoint their situation via satellite signals. In mountainous terrain an altimeter is also a useful aid to navigation.

Rock climbing, snow and ice mountaineering and glacier travel all require specific expertise, and skills may vary depending on the type and difficulty of the objective. Recognizing approaching adverse weather and avoiding dangerous snow conditions and avalanche-prone slopes can facilitate safe passage in the mountains, but are skills which can only be refined over many years. All members of parties crossing where there is avalanche danger should carry an avalanche transceiver.

In more remote settings, rescue and evacuation plans should be made before they are needed. This task often falls to the expedition doctor. Communications lines to the local authorities should be investigated and formalized in advance. Two-way radio sets or satellite telephones should be considered when assistance might otherwise be delayed for more than 24 hours. In addition, when there is a casualty at a site remote from the expedition doctor, this equipment allows communication with the doctor at base camp. In Europe and North America, the use of digital portable telephones by climbers and skiers allows rescue by helicopter within minutes and could be considered essential safety equipment.

Travel health insurance often excludes climbing or winter sports. Helicopter rescue is very expensive. Travel agents should be able to advise about insurance, and in the UK the British Mountaineering Council offers advice and competitive cover (*see* Appendix 8, Useful addresses).

Courses

Numerous courses are advertised in outdoor, backpacking, climbing and mountaineering magazines (e.g. *High Mountain Sports*, Greenshires Print, Northants; *Climber*, Warners Group Holdings plc, Bourne, Lincs) which are available in many newsagents and outdoor equipment shops (also *see* Further reading).

Basic life support and first aid on mountains

Injuries are inevitable in an adventurous and unpredictable sport such as mountaineering. Trekkers and fell-walkers are also at risk from objective dangers such as rockfall and avalanche, and from unexpected medical emergencies such as myocardial infarction. Fortunately, first-aid techniques are the same on mountains as they are at the roadside. In most situations in Europe and North America where rescue is near at hand, basic first aid will ensure that the injured or sick individual survives the wait for the rescue services. Individuals seeking travel advice could be encouraged to attend a first-aid course.

A brief summary of basic life support/first-aid measures is given below and expanded as an algorithm on page 117, which may guide doctors in directing their patients.

1   Ensure that the rescuer and the victim are safe from further danger.

2   Demonstrate unresponsiveness (check response to voice and, if no response, to pain).

3   Airway – ensure that airway is clear from obstruction, lift chin and tilt head backwards. Immobilize cervical spine if trauma is suspected and open the airway by jaw thrust manoeuvre instead.

4   Breathing – observe for spontaneous breathing. If absent, and after checking pulse, commence artificial respiration (12 breaths per minute in an adult, 20 breaths per minute in a child).

5   Circulation – check carotid pulse. If absent, commence cardiac massage at a rate of 100 chest compressions per minute in an adult or a child (15 chest compressions:2 breaths in an adult, 5:1 in a child).

6   Bleeding – direct pressure to bleeding point and elevate.

7   Recovery position – in the unconscious patient who is breathing spontaneously. Keep back and neck straight if there is a risk of spinal injury.

8   Fractures – splint to prevent movement, elevate to reduce swelling and cover compound fractures with a clean dressing. Splints can be improvised from skis, ice axes, rucksack frames, rolled-up sleeping mat, trees, tent poles, etc. Legs can be splinted to the uninjured contralateral limb and upper arm injuries managed in a sling. Lower arm injuries should be splinted. Keep back and neck straight if there is any suggestion of spinal or head injury. Improvise a collar for neck injuries (use sleeping mat, folded newspaper, etc.).

9   Hypothermia and avalanche – *see* Chapter 5.

10   Frostbite – *see* Chapter 5.

11   Overheating – *see* Chapter 5.

12   Near drowning – prolonged resuscitation.

Box 9.1: Basic life support

A Airway maintenance and cervical spine control
B Breathing and ventilation
C Circulation and haemorrhage control
D Disability: neurological status
E Exposure/environment control (core temperature)

Medical emergencies in accessible and in remote places

As increasing numbers of individuals from all walks of life, of all ages and levels of fitness choose to spend their leisure time on mountains and in remote wildernesses, the chance that medical emergencies will occur is rising. In one study of trekking deaths, 10% of trekkers who died were thought to have suffered myocardial infarction and 8% diabetic keto-acidosis. In a remote place, the location, skills in the party and available equipment will determine what can be done when a member becomes ill.

Cardiac arrest following injury or myocardial infarction should initially be managed by attempted cardiopulmonary resuscitation along the lines described previously (*see* Figure 9.1). At altitude, or on mountains where there is danger from avalanche, rockfall or steepness of the slope, attempts at resuscitation should not be undertaken if there will be a danger to the safety of those first on the scene. If there is a likelihood of rapid rescue, cardiopulmonary resuscitation (CPR) should be continued until the rescue services arrive. CPR is exhausting, and should be undertaken by as many people as possible in a safe site. Where there is no response to initial resuscitative attempts and no hope of rescue within a few hours, it is reasonable to discontinue after one hour. If the victim has hypothermia, prolonged resuscitation should be considered (*see* Chapter 5).

Myocardial ischaemia, angina and heart failure should be treated as at sea level, but oxygen and descent are important adjuncts to treatment at altitude. Stroke and other acute neurological events should also be managed as at sea level. Descent and administration of oxygen are helpful,

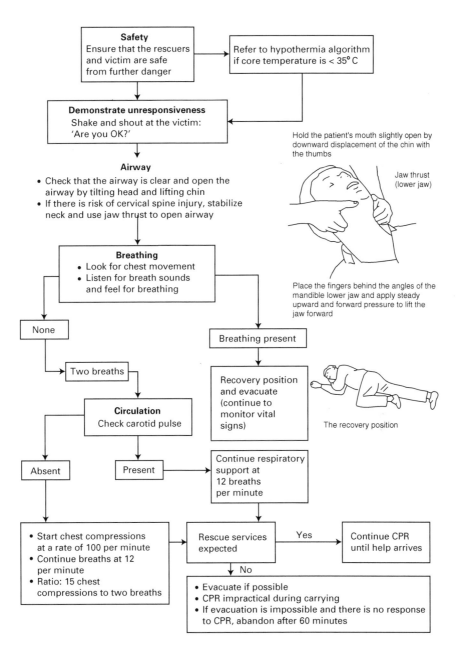

Safety
Ensure that the rescuers and victim are safe from further danger

Refer to hypothermia algorithm if core temperature is < 35° C

Demonstrate unresponsiveness
Shake and shout at the victim: 'Are you OK?'

Hold the patient's mouth slightly open by downward displacement of the chin with the thumbs

Airway
- Check that the airway is clear and open the airway by tilting head and lifting chin
- If there is risk of cervical spine injury, stabilize neck and use jaw thrust to open airway

Jaw thrust (lower jaw)

Breathing
- Look for chest movement
- Listen for breath sounds and feel for breathing

Place the fingers behind the angles of the mandible lower jaw and apply steady upward and forward pressure to lift the jaw forward

None

Breathing present

Two breaths

Recovery position and evacuate (continue to monitor vital signs)

The recovery position

Circulation
Check carotid pulse

Absent

Present

Continue respiratory support at 12 breaths per minute

- Start chest compressions at a rate of 100 per minute
- Continue breaths at 12 per minute
- Ratio: 15 chest compressions to two breaths

Rescue services expected

Yes

Continue CPR until help arrives

No

- Evacuate if possible
- CPR impractical during carrying
- If evacuation is impossible and there is no response to CPR, abandon after 60 minutes

Figure 9.1: Basic life support algorithm (Handley *et al.*, 1997; Resuscitation Council (UK), 2000; Colquhoun *et al.*, 2003).

and vital when the neurological event is associated with altitude itself (*see* Chapter 3). Acute asthma, pneumonia and other acute respiratory illnesses should be managed with oxygen and descent when possible, in addition to standard therapies such as bronchodilators for asthma and antibiotics for pneumonia.

Buried avalanche victims may be asphyxiated. If there is an air pocket, the victim may survive for some time before running out of oxygen. Resuscitation should be attempted in an apnoeic victim, as respiratory arrest may have only just occurred (*see* Chapter 5).

Most other medical emergencies are relatively unaffected by altitude, but may become all the more serious on a mountainside in the absence of diagnostic and therapeutic tools. The use of common sense, accepting limitations of equipment and drugs, and improvisation are the keys to management of medical emergencies. In the unconscious patient, fluids can be given rectally if facilities for safe administration by alternative routes are unavailable.

Remote surgery

Surgical emergencies in a remote environment should be managed conservatively whenever possible, and evacuation undertaken immediately.

When the presentation is with abdominal pain, the possibility of medical illness should be considered (tropical infections, gastroenteritis, urinary tract infection, myocardial infarction, diabetes). The acute abdomen should be managed with antibiotics and analgesia if the patient is stable (diverticulitis, cholecystitis, salpingitis, appendicitis, colic, pancreatitis). Surgery may be required later (to drain a collection of pus), but should only be undertaken in the field if the patient is deteriorating and there is little hope of rescue.

Rupture of a viscus (spleen, aorta, ectopic pregnancy) is likely to present with shock, may be rapidly fatal and will require surgical expertise for management. Bowel perforation (appendix, diverticulum, peptic ulcer) should be managed conservatively with antibiotics and analgesia except in a shocked or deteriorating patient, and where surgical expertise and equipment are available. Bowel obstruction should be managed conservatively with a nasogastric tube (may be improvised from a urinary catheter) on intermittent suction (with a syringe) and free drainage. There is a danger of dehydration, and intravenous or rectal fluids should be administered.

Some surgical conditions, such as abscesses, can be treated under local anaesthesia. Such minor surgery may facilitate evacuation. No surgery which could be performed electively should be undertaken in the field, because of the risks of anaesthesia and surgery and their complications.

Anaesthesia at altitude

There is little likelihood of appropriate equipment or expertise being available for general anaesthesia at high altitude. There are particular dangers from unpredictable performance of the anaesthetic machine and intra-operative hypoxia at low environmental pressure. The principles of safe anaesthesia at high altitude are discussed in detail by Stoneham (1995). With due attention to oxygenation, anaesthesia seems relatively safe up to 3500 m. Whenever possible, general anaesthesia should be avoided at very high altitude (particularly above 4000 m). In this situation anaesthesia, if absolutely essential, should be with a volatile agent (such as halothane or isoflurane) in 100% oxygen (Stoneham, 1995). Local anaesthesia is pre-ferred whenever possible.

When surgery is required, but evacuation is impossible and local anaesthesia is impractical, the use of ketamine is the safest option (Bishop *et al.*, 2000). The airway is usually maintained by the patient under ketamine anaesthesia, but should still be monitored. Hypoxia does occur with ketamine anaesthesia at altitude, and oxygen should be admin-istered if possible. Hallucinations and transient psychosis may occur (less commonly in children), and may be controlled by premedication with a benzodiazepine.

Orthopaedics and trauma on mountains

Some 30% of trekker deaths in Nepal result from trauma, and 35% die of altitude related illness (Shlim and Gallie, 1992). Among British climbers on peaks over 7000 m, some 70% of deaths were caused by falls, rockfall or avalanche (Pollard and Clarke, 1988). The management of orthopaedic injuries in the mountains consists primarily of first-aid measures and evacuation, but particular attention to oxygenation and prevention of hypothermia are necessary.

Climbers with head injuries should be evacuated as rapidly as possible. The cervical spine should be immobilized. Basic first-aid measures, airway, breathing and circulation (ABC), should be undertaken, a survey of head, neck, chest, abdomen, pelvis, spine and extremities made to exclude other injuries, and a conservative observational approach used. The conscious level, pulse (and blood pressure when available), respiratory rate and pupils should be monitored. When the neurological condition is rapidly deteriorating and there is a suspicion of intracranial haematoma (extra/subdural), surgery has been advocated by some who have had good results. However, it would be unusual for the necessary neurosurgical equipment for drilling burr holes and expertise to be available in the field. Use of dexamethasone and mannitol (if available) could be considered to reduce associated cerebral oedema. Bladder catheterization would normally be required prior to administration of mannitol. As an alternative to urethral catheterization, an intravenous cannula may be used to drain the bladder suprapubically. Possible skull fractures should be treated with antibiotics if there is evidence of a compound fracture indicated by cerebrospinal fluid (CSF) leakage from ears or nose or lacerations to the skin of the head. Non-sedative drugs are preferred for analgesia to ensure that the patient continues to maintain his own airway and to facilitate monitoring of changes in neurological status during evacuation. Oxygen should be administered if it is available.

It should be assumed that the neck has been injured if there has been a fall. Management involves splinting the neck using an improvised cervical collar. In an unconscious patient, a collar should remain *in situ* during evacuation. In a conscious patient, management of the neck injury can be reassessed after examination of the neck and neurological examination.

When limb fractures and dislocations occur in mountain resorts, first-aid measures to splint the limb and provide analgesia should be undertaken until evacuation to hospital can be achieved. In a remote setting, attention to blood supply and neurological function below the fracture and analgesia are of prime importance. In both upper and lower limb fractures, arterial pulsations distal to the fracture should be sought. If these are absent, the limb may be lost. Attempts to re-align the bones or reduce the dislocation should be made to restore blood supply and to facilitate evacuation and splinting. If any manoeuvre results in the loss of peripheral arterial pulsation, the manoeuvre should be reversed. Fractures may place tension on the overlying skin which would undergo necrosis if not relieved. Also in this situation reduction of a fracture should be considered. Once a compound fracture has been reduced and the blood supply is intact, the biggest threat to the limb is from infection. Antibiotics should be administered until wound toilet in hospital is available.

Chest injuries should be managed conservatively with adequate analgesia to facilitate coughing and evacuation. Flail chest is managed with analgesia, and intercostal nerve block might be considered if skills are available. The possibility of pneumothorax should always be considered and must be drained if under tension. A degree of improvisation may be required, and a Heimlich valve is more practical than an under-water drain.

In competitive sport climbing, upper limb injuries other than fractures are particularly common (Bollen, 1990). The most common injuries described are A2 pulley injury of the finger (damage to the flexor sheath of the flexor digitorum superficialis tendon at the base of the proximal phalanx causing 'bowstringing' of the flexor tendon), fixed flexion deformity of the fingers, brachialis tendinitis at the elbow, medial and lateral epicondylitis at the elbow, and impingement syndrome at the shoulder.

Remote dentistry

Avoiding dental problems at high altitude

The best advice is to leave dental problems at home. A thorough dental examination, including a panoramic X-ray, is recommended at least four months prior to departure. The dentist should be invited to attend to all problems and potential problems that might otherwise spoil the trip. Toothache ranks with renal colic as one of the most consistently distracting pains. Treatment may take months for the dentist to achieve. Consequently, time should be allowed to ensure that all symptoms have been successfully treated well in advance of departure.

Common dental problems on expeditions

Teeth that react to cold or hot stimuli (decay cavities, leaking fillings and broken teeth) will be uncomfortable in cold climates. The custom of loading one's diet with sugary carbohydrates at altitude is common, and it must be remembered that this diet will cause rapid dental decay. While changes in barometric pressure can greatly trouble divers and pilots with dental problems, the same does not seem to occur in travellers at high altitude.

The incidence of those with wisdom teeth (third molar) problems increases in the 18–25 years age group. Many of this age range travel to high altitude. While living in high camps, few would disagree that some compromise in personal habits can occur. Oral anaerobic bacteria thrive around third molars in such circumstances, particularly when fed on a diet of refined carbohydrates. The resulting infection and swelling can be dramatic and uncomfortable, and can spread throughout the oral soft tissues.

Dental first-aid kit

It is appropriate to use *surgical gloves* for all dental procedures.

2 dental mirrors, 1 probe, for diagnosis.

1 pair locking tweezers, for use with *cotton wool* to dry cavities prior to placing a dressing.

Cotton wool rolls for control of saliva and haemorrhage.

1 flat-bladed instrument for placing dressings.

1 spatula and mixing slab for mixing temporary dressings.

1 fine Spencer Wells forceps, black silk thread on fine semi-lunar needle.

Fine curved scissors for placing sutures.

1 local anaesthetic syringe, local anaesthetic cartridges.

Extraction forceps are best carried only by the experienced.

Antibiotics. Amoxycillin/clavulanic acid 500 mg, erythromycin 500 mg, metronidazole 200 mg. Antibiotic allergies and sensitivities should be identified before departure.

Pain relief. Ibuprofen 400 mg, clove oil.

Learning how to perform basic dental block anaesthesia may prove useful to expedition doctors (*see* Tables 9.1 and 9.2).

Table 9.1: Some basic symptoms, diagnoses and treatments for damaged teeth

Symptom	Diagnosis	Treatment
Pain with hot, cold, sweet stimulus	Cavity or inadequate filling	Place temporary filling into dry cavity
Severe pain with hot, cold stimulus; prolonged ache; unable to sleep because of pain	Deep cavity or filling causing continual dental nerve irritation	Place temporary filling; antibiotics, e.g. amoxycillin/clavulanic acid (500 mg tds); ibuprofen (400 mg, max. six/day)
Acute swelling and toothache; continual ache; unable to sleep	Serious infection/ abscess	Broad-spectrum antibiotic, e.g. amoxycillin/clavulanic acid (500 mg tds 1/52); metronidazole (200 mg tds 1/52); ibuprofen (400 mg, max. six/day)
Persistence of symptoms despite antibiotic treatment	Irreversible infection	Extraction or root treatment required; refer and evacuate to expert care
Gum infections and severe bleeding	Poor oral hygiene; vitamin deficiency	Hot concentrated salty water as mouthwash; metronidazole (200 mg qds 4/7); vitamin supplements

Table 9.2:   Serious dental trauma
(this could be caused by a climbing fall, falling rock or ice, or avalanche)

Symptom	Diagnosis	Treatment
Broken teeth with no bleeding visible from within the tooth structure	Fracture of enamel and dentine	Temporarily dress if possible; check lip lacerations for tooth fragments
Broken teeth with bleeding from internal tooth structure	Fracture exposing dental nerve and blood vessels	Antibiotic and pain relief; do not temporarily dress; check lip lacerations for tooth fragments; seek immediate expert care
Teeth that have been moved with associated minor bone fractures	Saveable teeth	Reposition teeth using finger strength; antibiotics and pain relief; seek immediate expert care
Teeth that have been knocked out in their entirety	Less than 45% saveable	If clean, reposition into socket with finger strength immediately. If possible in less than 30 minutes clean with sterile saline. Give antibiotics and pain relief. If unable to replant, transport tooth in saline, milk or saliva – do not allow to dry out. Seek dental advice urgently
Fracture to zygomatic arch or mandible	Serious injury, including shock	Arrest any haemorrhage; pain relief; vertical support bandaging; high-calorie soft diet; seek immediate expert care

Temporary dressings for damaged teeth

These come in two forms. Premixed paste is the easiest to use and can be extruded from a tube. It is fairly soft, but erodes relatively quickly. There are a variety of proprietary brands (e.g. Cavit by ESPE). Less easy to use but recommended is a material called 'IRM', as it is an intermediate restorative material (Dentsply). It was developed for use in Vietnam and originally coloured red, blue and white, depending on the priority for further treatment. The white version, which is widely available, presents as a powder and liquid for mixing into a thick putty. It sets quickly, and is durable for at least a year if placed into a dry and retentive shaped cavity.

These materials are available from the Dental Directory, Billericay Dental Supply Co. Ltd, 6 Perry Way, Wiltham, Essex CM8 3SX (Tel: 0800 585 586).

References and further reading

Mountain skills, communications and mountain rescue

Books
Cliff P (1991) *Mountain Navigation*. Published by P Cliff.

Langmuir E (1995) *Mountaincraft and Leadership*. Scottish Sports Council, Edinburgh.

March B (1982) *Modern Rope Techniques in Mountaineering*. Cicerone, Milnthorne.

March B (1988) *Modern Snow and Ice Techniques*. Cicerone, Milnthorne.

Courses
British Mountain Guides, Capel Curig, Gwynedd, North Wales LL24 0ET. Website: bmg@mltb.org

International School of Mountaineering, Switzerland. UK enquiries to Hafod Tan-Y-Graig, Nant Gwynant, Gwynedd LL55 4NW. Tel: 01766 890441. Fax: 01766 890599. Website: ism@alpin-ism.com

The National Mountain Centre, Plas Y Brenin, Capel Curig, Gwynedd LL24 0ET. Tel: 01690 720214.

The Outward Bound Trust, 207 Waterloo Road, London SE1 8XD. Tel: 0870 5134227. Email: enquiries@outwardbound-uk.org

The Scottish National Sports Centre, Glenmore Lodge, Aviemore, Inverness-shire PH22 1QU. Tel: 01479 861276.

Basic life support and first aid on mountains

Books for the general public
Duff J and Gormly P (2001) *First Aid and Survival in Mountain and Remote Areas*. Cordee, Leicester.

St John Ambulance, St Andrew's Ambulance Association and the British Red Cross Society (2002) *First Aid Manual* (8e). Dorling Kindersley, London.

Steele P (1999) *Medical Handbook for Walkers and Climbers (A Constable Guide)*. Constable Robinson, London.

Information for doctors
Colquhoun MC, Handley AJ and Evans TR (eds) (2003) *ABC of Resuscitation*. BMJ Books, London.

Handley AJ, Becker LB, Allen M *et al*. (1997) Single-rescuer adult basic life support: an advisory statement from the Basic Life Support Working Group of the International Liaison Committee on Resuscitation. *Circulation*. **95**: 2174–9.

Resuscitation Council (UK) (2000) *Resuscitation Guidelines for Use in the UK*. Resuscitation Council (UK), London.

Resuscitation Council (2002) *Advanced Life Support Manual* (4e). Resuscitation Council UK Trading Ltd, London.

Courses for doctors
British Association for Immediate Care (BASICS), Turret House, Turret Lane, Ipswich IP4 1DL. Tel: 0870 1654999. Fax: 0870 1654949. Email: admin@basics.org.uk

Anaesthesia at altitude

Bishop RA, Litch JA and Stanton JM (2000) Ketamine anesthesia at high altitude. *High Alt Med Biol*. **1**: 111–14.

Stoneham MD (1995) Anaesthesia and resuscitation at altitude. *Eur J Anaesthesiol*. **12**: 249–57.

Orthopaedics and trauma

Bollen SR (1990) Upper limb injuries in elite rock climbers. *J R Coll Surg Edinb*. **35**: 18–20.

Bollen SR and Wright V (1994) Radiographic changes in the hands of rock climbers. *Br J Sports Med*. **28**: 185–6.

Bowie WS, Hunt TK and Allen HA (1988) Rock-climbing injuries in Yosemite National Park. *West J Med*. **149**: 172–7.

Haas JC and Meyers MC (1995) Rock climbing injuries. *Sports Med*. **20**: 199–205.

Limb D (1995) Injuries on British climbing walls. *Br J Sports Med*. **29**: 168–70.

Peters P (2001) Orthopedic problems in sport climbing. *Wild Environ Med*. **12**: 100–10.

Pollard AJ and Clarke C (1988) Deaths during mountaineering at extreme altitude. *Lancet*. **i**: 1277.

Shlim DR and Gallie J (1992) The causes of death among trekkers in Nepal. *Int J Sports Med*. **13**: 74–6.

Villar RN (1986) Casualties on Everest – an evacuation problem. *Injury*. **17**: 138–42.

Remote dentistry

Andreason FM and Daugaard-Jensen J (1991) Treatment of traumatic dental injuries in children. *Curr Opin Dent*. **5**: 535–50.

Blinkhorn AS and Mackie IC (1996) My child's just knocked out a front tooth. *BMJ*. **32**: 526.

Mackie IC and Worthington HV (1992) An investigation of replantation of traumatically avulsed permanent incisor teeth. *Br Dent J*. **172**: 17–20.

Newton CW (1992) Trauma involving the dentition and supporting tissues. *Curr Opin Dent*. **2**: 108–14.

10

Health, environment and local culture

Water disinfection

Ensuring that water is not contaminated is an important part of pre-ventative medicine on a trek or expedition. The expedition or trek doctor should take a lead role in inspecting water sources and ensuring that latrines are placed away from this site.

There are several methods of field water disinfection:

1 heat

2 filtration

3 clarification

4 chemical disinfection.

Heat

Boiling is the most effective method for sterilizing water. It kills all enteric pathogens, including bacteria, viruses and protozoa. Boiling water vigor-ously for at least one minute is sufficient, even at high altitudes. This treatment is not affected by the chemical composition of the water or the presence of sediment. Unfortunately, boiling may not always be practical because of technical, fuel or time constraints.

Filtration

Filtration will remove bacteria, protozoal cysts and parasitic eggs, but will not adequately remove viruses. Most commercially available filters claim to remove bacteria and *Giardia*. Some incorporate halogen resins or activated charcoal to further aid disinfection.

Clarification

Clarification techniques such as sedimentation, flocculation and charcoal filters are not sufficient to disinfect water, but may be used to remove organic matter prior to filtration or chemical disinfection.

Chemical disinfection

Chlorine and iodine are the most widely used chemical disinfectants. They are effective against viruses, bacteria and protozoal cysts. Iodine has the advantage of being more effective against protozoal cysts, and is more palatable than chlorine. Both halogens react with organic impurities in the water, and thus particulate matter should be removed by filtration, sedimentation or other techniques before treatment. The effectiveness of halogen disinfection depends on the water temperature, concentration of the halogen and contact time of the halogen with the water. Cold water and lower halogen concentrations require a longer time before the water is safe to consume. Any flavouring should be added to the water after sufficient contact time.

Iodine may be best avoided in those with uncontrolled thyroid disorders and those with iodine allergy.

There are various techniques for disinfection of water with chlorine and iodine. Both chlorine- and iodine-based tablets are commercially available and, when using them, the manufacturer's instructions should be followed. The Wilderness Medical Society (Forgey, 1995) recommends halogen doses (per litre of water) and contact times for various water temperatures (*see* Tables 10.1 and 10.2).

Sustainable trekking

In recent years there has been an increased awareness of the impact of tourism on developing countries. A responsible approach to the environmental and cultural effects of trekking and mountaineering in developing

Table 10.1: Chemical disinfection: recommended halogen doses per litre of water

Halogenation technique	Amount per litre for 4 parts per million (ppm)
Tetraglycine hydroperiodide tablets	½ tablet
2% iodine solution (tincture)	0.2 ml, 5 drops
10% povidone-iodine solution	0.35 ml, 8 drops
Saturated iodine crystals in water	14 ml
Saturated iodine crystals in alcohol	0.1 ml for 5 ppm
Halazone tablets (mono-dichloraminobenzoic acid)	2 tablets
Household bleach 5% (sodium hypochlorite)	0.1 ml, 2 drops

Table 10.2: Chemical disinfection: recommended contact time for halogen and various water temperatures

Concentration of halogen (ppm)	Contact time (minutes)		
	5°C	15°C	30°C
4	180	60	45
8	60	30	15

countries prior to travel may reduce some of the adverse consequences of tourism and enhance the benefits.

The philosophy which encompasses current thinking on these issues is known as 'sustainable development' which, according to the most widely acknowledged definition:

meets the needs of the present without compromising the ability of future generations to meet their own needs.
(World Commission on Environment and Development, 1987)

Trekking and mountaineering can be considered in this context, and a trek or expedition doctor might wish to consider his or her role in promoting sustainable development.

Benefits of tourism

For the individual trekker there are benefits in cultural exchange, aesthetic appreciation of the natural world and self-fulfilment in completing the physical challenge of a trek or climb. For industrialized nations, the developing world may be viewed as a resource for 'primary' products (including new food sources, medicines, etc.), an assimilative capacity to absorb wastes, and a life support service for maintaining complex systems such as the atmosphere. For the developing country there may be economic advantages of tourism and employment opportunities for local inhabitants in addition to beneficial cultural exchange.

Disadvantages of tourism

On the other hand, an influx of tourists may encourage deforestation through an increased use of wood for fuel and building, pollution with non-biodegradable packaging and exhaust from fuel, pollution of water sources from inadequate provision of sanitation, economic reliance (loss of traditional skills such as farming), erosion of soil and vegetation on popular trekking routes, economic inequality and adverse cultural exchange.

Reducing the impact of tourism

Packaging and solid waste. Where possible avoid plastics. Use paper and other biodegradable packaging. Burn all solid waste or remove it to local facilities/country of origin for incineration.

Batteries. Remove all batteries to country of origin for incineration. Batteries are a hazard to the environment from leaching of chemicals, and are a danger to animals and children following ingestion.

Fuel. Avoid using wood as a fuel. Consider using solar power or micro-hydro energy for large expeditions. Gas and liquid fuels are the most commonly used, and although they deplete resources, the amount used by a trekking group is insignificant in comparison to use by industrialized nations. The greatest environmental impact of fuel use is from the spent aviation fuel in reaching the destination.

Culture. Respect local customs and culture by supporting and understanding cultural differences.

Health. Support local health systems by avoiding inappropriate treatment of locals (see below).

Human waste disposal

Where possible, trekking groups in developing countries should dig latrines to accommodate their waste, as the facilities used by local inhabitants will not usually have the necessary capacity. Latrines should be placed well away from water sources in order to avoid contamination. The trek doctor should oversee sanitation and educate all members of the group, especially the cook, in the prevention of infection.

When it is not possible to dig latrines because the ground is too rocky, frozen or is the unyielding ice of a glacier, then alternative strategies are required. One method is to dry the faeces in a 25-mm-thick layer in the sun, which massively reduces bulk (by 40% in 60 hours and 60% in 140 hours at Everest Base Camp in September) and smell. Turning of the faecal solids and shielding from rain will aid drying. The desiccated faeces may then be burned, removed for use as fertilizer or incinerated where facilities are available. Defaecation in privacy should be encouraged, but disposal of human waste behind a rock, in the shade, will prolong pollution of the area and pose a health hazard. All toilet paper should be burned.

Medical treatment of local people

Travellers to developing countries are often approached by locals requesting medical assistance. The appropriate response is not always easy to determine. In most cases the best approach is to refer them to the local health facility and not to dispense medications. It is highly unlikely that travelling health professionals will be able to significantly benefit those with chronic diseases, minor complaints and many acute illnesses. Indeed, by freely dispensing medications the traveller reinforces the notion that foreign medicine is superior, and runs the risk of eroding confidence in local health services. To make matters worse, foreign medications are usually more colourful and attractive than those produced in the developing world, and are consequently considered to be more potent. On the other hand, confidence in Western medicine may be lost by inadequate or inappropriate therapy. Only initiate therapies that will work, and avoid the temptation to use placebos. This approach may seem harsh, but it is ultimately in the best interests of the individual and the country.

In some situations it is clearly appropriate to offer what medical assistance you can confidently manage (e.g. assisting someone injured). The health of local guides, porters, cooks and other staff in your employ is to a large degree your responsibility. They should receive the same medical attention as other travellers in the expedition, and should never be abandoned when unwell.

References and further reading

Backer HD (1995) Field water disinfection. In: PA Auerbach (ed.) *Wilderness Medicine: management of wilderness and environmental emergencies.* Mosby-Year Book, St Louis, MO, pp. 1060–110.

Backer H (2002) Water disinfection for international and wilderness travelers. *Clin Infect Dis.* **34**: 355–64.

Bezruchka S (1992) Medical treatment of local people by travelers. *J Wilderness Med.* **3**: 1–3.

Bishop RA and Litch JA (2000) Medical tourism can do harm. *BMJ.* **320**: 1017.

Forgey WW (1995) *Wilderness Medical Society Practice Guidelines for Wilderness Emergency Care.* ICS Books, Merrillville, IN.

Useful organization

The International Porter Protection Group. Website: www.ippg.net

11

Medico–legal considerations for treks and expeditions

Introduction

Expeditions offer an exciting challenge to the expedition medical officer. While their role is key to the success of an expedition, medical officers may find themselves liable for the care that they give if it is deemed to be inadequate or incorrect.

Cases in which a doctor is sued for treatment given on an expedition have not been noted in the UK. The fact that society is becoming more litigious has been highlighted by the case of the action *Woodroffe Hedley v Cuthbertson*, in which the English High Court, in June 1997, found against Dave Cuthbertson, a climbing guide who had been sued by his client's widow arising out of an accident on a climbing trip in France, so it is an issue that must be looked at very seriously. On 15 June 2003 the *Sunday Times* newspaper reported that the family of Michael Matthews reached an out-of-court settlement at the High Court in Birmingham, UK, with £70 000 in damages being agreed. He was the youngest British person to climb Everest in 1999 but died on the descent whilst allegedly using faulty oxygen equipment. The limited company, the director, the guide and the supplier of the oxygen were all sued.

Insurance will not remove the risk of being sued, but certainly it should give peace of mind. All doctors should check the nature of their medical protection cover prior to embarking on a trip. For example, since October 1999, the Medical Defence Union has provided Good Samaritan cover for the whole of the world (the USA and Canada having previously been excepted).

Duty of care

In any potential court action, a duty of care must be established between the person giving the treatment and the patient. Clearly, if any doctor treats a patient, whether as a trek/expedition doctor (i.e. one of his charges) or in a rescue situation, it will be established. A duty of care, it must be remembered, is not owed to the world at large, but to those to whom injury may reasonably and probably be anticipated if the duty is not observed. It must be remembered that a doctor giving advice to a trekking company is clearly caught by this and owes a duty of care to the trekkers, even though he has never actually seen them.

Standard of care

One then moves on to consider what the standard of care is. In England, the matter is governed by the court's decision in *Bolam v Friern Hospital Management Committee* [1957] 1WLR 582, in which it is stated that 'The test is the standard of the ordinary skilled man exercising and professing to have that special skill. A man need not possess the highest expert skill at the risk of being found negligent. It is well established that it is sufficient, if he exercises the ordinary skill of an ordinary competent man exercising that particular art.'

Clearly, then, any person who is an actual expedition doctor will have to exercise the standard of care to be expected of an expedition doctor, and a doctor cannot plead (in essence) inexperience.

Inexperience

The law requires the trainee or learner to be judged by the same standard as his more experienced colleagues. If it did not, inexperience would frequently be urged as a defence to an action of professional negligence. If the defendant cannot exercise reasonable care, he should not undertake the task at all. A doctor who holds himself to be a specialist (i.e. for the purposes of this chapter, an expedition doctor) will be held to the standards of a reasonably competent expedition doctor even if he is a novice, and even where he is performing the procedure for the first time.

In a well-known case called *Nettleship v Weston* [1971] 2QB 691, Lord Denning, in the Court of Appeal, in a case which albeit was dealing with a learner driver, stated that 'The learner driver may be doing his best, but his incompetent best is not good enough.' He also stated that 'It is no answer for the driver to say "I was a learner driver under instruction. I was doing my best and could not help it". Civil law permits no such excuse.' This principle applies with as much force to an inexperienced doctor as it does to an inexperienced motorist. In *Jones v Manchester Corporation* [1952] 2AER 125, a patient died from an excessive dose of anaesthetic which had been administered by a doctor who had been qualified for 5 months. Again, in the Court of Appeal, Lord Denning said 'Error due to inexperience or lack of supervision are no defence as against the injured person' (see also the Court of Appeal comments in the recent case of *Wilsher v Essex Area Health Authority* [1986] 3AER 801).

Emergencies

What an expedition doctor is most probably going to be facing is what could be described as an emergency situation, and in determining what is reasonable care, the court will take account of the particular situation as it presented itself to the defendant as part and parcel of all the circumstances of the case. Clearly the court would take into account the fact that one is in a remote area and one's resources would be limited (one is not in an Accident and Emergency unit). This is highlighted by one of the judge's comments in the case of *Wilsher*, where it is stated 'Again I accept that full allowance must be made to the fact that certain aspects of treatment may have to be carried out in what one witness called "battle conditions". An emergency may overburden the available resources, and if an individual is forced by circumstances to do too many things, the fact that he does one of them incorrectly should not lightly be taken as negligence.'

Expectations of expedition members

Expedition members should not expect to receive the same standard of care that they would be given in a hospital casualty department, but should expect to receive a similar standard to that provided by any competent doctor in a similar situation. It is useful for an expedition medical officer to discuss prior to the expedition, with the expedition members, what standard of care the latter can expect to receive given the limitations of the expedition environment. He should also ask members to fill out a relevant health questionnaire.

Different opinions

In the context of standard of care, where different opinions exist about the acceptability of a course of conduct, if a doctor can show that the course he followed was one which has the backing of a body of respectable opinion within the profession, then liability will not be imposed merely because the treatment may be disproved by a section of medical opinion. Thus if one is able to obtain support from various doctors or organizations involved in expedition medicine, organization of courses in expedition medicine, or publishing relevant books or protocols (such as that laid out in the *British Antarctic Survey Medical Handbook*), one is well on the way to protecting any doctor and paramedic or trek leader (see *Bolitho v Hackney Health Authority* [1997] 4AER 771).

Trek leader/paramedic

Clearly the standard of care provided by a paramedic is not that of a doctor, but rather the standard of an ordinary skilled paramedic professing to have the special skill of a paramedic. The trek leader would likewise have to exercise the standard of skill expected of a trek leader.

Trek/expedition doctor/ Good Samaritan Act

Generally speaking, if one was travelling as a trek/expedition doctor, even if there was no payment for one's services, there would be no Good Samaritan cover. Quite often a doctor will not be paid *per se* but will receive a discount or some other benefit. In general, Good Samaritan cover is really only available if one is there as an ordinary person (i.e. as a layman) and not as a doctor, and one decides to deal with someone in one's party, or one deals with someone who is completely unconnected with one's expedition. Obviously if one is acting under the auspices of a Good Samaritan, the standard of care will only be that of what is expected from a normal GP (if one happens to be a GP).

Clearly if anyone is going on an expedition as a trek/expedition doctor, there should be a pre-trek/expedition questionnaire for all members of the party, and one must be absolutely certain that they are competent.

Trekking company/appointment of doctor

There is a duty on the part of the trekking company to appoint a competent doctor if they are appointing one at all. As a trekking company, they should check the doctor's experience. A normal GP with no experience would be risky, and in general the trek company will always be liable for the actions of the doctor. Even if the doctor is held to be an independent contractor, he is usually still under the control of the company and they will be responsible for his actions.

Can a doctor avoid liability by disclaimers?

Arguably if the doctor is not being paid and he persuaded each and every trekker to sign a disclaimer of liability prior to giving treatment, he might avoid liability. Generally speaking such disclaimers are caught by the Unfair Contract Terms Act 1977 (As Amended). Equally, trekking companies sometimes try to persuade clients to sign disclaimers, but these are caught by the Act, as the latter applies to anything arising in the course of business, and this is generally given a fairly broad meaning.

This should be compared with the position in America and Canada, where companies certainly can ask clients to sign disclaimers and, subject to them being written clearly and properly, these will be effective in absolving the companies of all liability for negligent acts, etc. (see the American case *Patricia Vodopest v Rosemary Macgregor*, Supreme Court of Washington, 8 March 1996 and the Canadian case known as *Bay Street Court Decision*, Supreme Court of British Columbia, 20 September 1996).

Advice and prescribing for trek leaders/ first aiders for the use of unknown third parties

Obviously the duty of care is not to the world at large, but to those to whom injury may reasonably and probably be anticipated. GPs giving advice to the above are caught fairly and squarely, and if they are going to do it, they should clearly label the drugs, and give indications of the use, contraindications, possible side-effects and how to administer the drugs. Clearly the person using the drug should then be knowledgeable.

The Crown Report (1999) recommends that prescription-only medication (POMs) when given by a person who is not registered as a medical practitioner should be governed by written and signed protocols. It is therefore advisable for any expedition medical officer who is not a doctor to have written and signed protocols for all expedition drugs.

Conclusion

Perhaps the most important thing of all is for anyone contemplating going on an expedition/trek as a doctor, paramedic/nurse, etc. to ensure that they have the appropriate insurance cover. This must be checked with the relevant professional bodies prior to departure.

Finally, if one is considering acting in any capacity other than as a Good Samaritan, one should be able to satisfy oneself that one is able to deal competently with any medical problems that arise.

One should also try to obtain a written letter of engagement, in essence from the organizers, setting out what one's duties are and what is expected of one, and who is in overall command (especially with regard to medical matters). In addition, one should make enquiries about the company/ organization that is appointing one with regard to their reputation/track record, so that one can make an informed judgement as to whether to accept an appointment.

The above is a very brief synopsis of some of the medico–legal issues involved in treks and expeditions and is by no means definitive or exhaustive. This is a complex subject, and clearly matters should be discussed before setting out with the relevant professional indemnity organizations and one's own legal advisers.

Appendix 1

High altitude medical kit

The composition of a medical kit is governed by many factors, not the least being the personal preference of expedition members. Other factors include the following.

1 *Destination* – the altitudes encountered, presence of endemic diseases and distance from medical assistance need to be considered.

2 *Duration of the expedition.*

3 *Number of expedition members* – including porters and other hired expedition staff.

4 *Medical training of expedition members* – the presence of health professionals may permit the use of specialized medications and equipment.

5 *Expectations of expedition members* – members of commercial expeditions may expect a certain degree of medical expertise to be present.

6 *Past medical history of expedition members* – certain medications will be required for individuals with chronic or recurrent medical problems.

7 *Bulk, weight and cost* – important considerations for any expedition gear. Medical kits can be very expensive to put together.

Medications

Simple analgesics and antimicrobial agents are the most commonly used drugs on many expeditions. Antidiarrhoeals and throat lozenges are also widely dispensed. Choosing drugs with more than one use (e.g. codeine for its analgesic, antitussive and antidiarrhoeal properties) can reduce bulk. The route of administration for each drug should also be considered. Intravenous preparations may freeze, and oral medications may be dangerous to administer to patients with decreased consciousness or who are vomiting (when the rectal route may be preferable).

Some drugs (e.g. analgesics, H$_2$ blockers, acyclovir, steroid creams and rehydration solutions) are available over the counter in many countries. In the UK, private prescriptions should be used for medications prescribed for use *in an emergency,* since it is illegal to use an NHS prescription for this purpose. When controlled drugs are to be carried for use in an emergency, a Home Office licence may be obtained in the UK which is issued to doctors on application to the Home Office Drugs Branch (*see* Appendix 8, Useful addresses). Although the licence is only valid in the UK, many countries will be prepared to accept it, and it may be carried by either doctors or the general public. Application should be made by a doctor and should include the following information: country of destination, dates of travel (depart and return) and drug details (including name of drug, strength, formulation and total quantity to be carried).

Diagnostic equipment

The diagnostic equipment carried, if any, depends on the experience of the expedition members. If a member has medical training, a stethoscope, sphygmomanometer and ophthalmoscope may be carried. A low-reading thermometer is useful in cases of suspected hypothermia. Pulse oximeters, although expensive, come in small sizes with rechargeable batteries and may be a useful adjunct to clinical acumen at high altitudes. When using pulse oximeters, it is important to be aware of the normal arterial oxygen saturation levels for the altitudes encountered (for comparison, *see* Figure 1.2). Pulse oximeters have only been validated from 80–100% saturation, and reliability of the algorithm below this cannot be guaranteed. In addition, peripheral vasoconstriction in cold weather may affect the accuracy of pulse oximeters. Lithium batteries weigh less, last longer and are more temperature tolerant than alkaline batteries, and thus have advantages for use with electrical diagnostic and other equipment used in the mountains. Wright peak flow meters under-read with increasing altitude (by 31% at 5300 m) (*see* page 81). Turbine spirometers, such as the fixed orifice Micro

Medical turbine microspirometer (Micro Medical, Rochester, Kent, UK) are unaffected by altitude.

Other equipment

Again, what is carried depends on the experience of expedition members, and may range from Steri-strips® for wound closure to sophisticated life support devices. A variety of lightweight and inflatable splints are available for orthopaedic injuries. Administration of intravenous fluids is usually impractical above base camp on a mountaineering expedition, largely due to difficulties keeping the fluids warm. Blood transfusion is almost always impractical in a wilderness setting.

Portable hyperbaric chamber

As mentioned previously, portable hyperbaric chambers can be a useful aid to facilitate descent (*see* page 22), but it remains a personal decision whether one is taken on an expedition. It is possible to hire them in some countries (e.g. Nepal). Purchase details can be found on page 33.

Containers for the medical kit

There are many types of containers that can be used for medical kits. Needless to say, whatever is chosen should provide protection from physical damage and temperature extremes, be lightweight and not bulky, be easily identified and allow ready access to its contents. Heavy-duty plastic barrels with a lockable lid are ideal. Security should also be considered as medicines are in short supply in developing countries, theft is common and many of the drugs carried are potentially dangerous.

Distribution of medical kits

On smaller expeditions, a small personal kit may be all that is required. On larger mountaineering expeditions, base camp kits and high altitude kits may be needed. The various kits should be sorted out and packed prior to departure.

An example of an expedition medical kit*

The kit outlined below attempts to provide a comprehensive list of items which, from the authors' experience, are likely to be required on an expedition to a high mountain when a doctor is present. This will need modification depending on the objective, experience of personnel, number of expedition members and finance. Additional drugs may be required for individuals with certain underlying conditions (e.g. heart failure, epilepsy, asthma). A simple personal kit can be carried by all expedition members.

Expedition kit (accompanied by a doctor)

All doses should be checked prior to usage with a standard formulary text. The doses quoted are for adults: im = intramuscular; iv = intravenous; qds = to be taken four times daily; tds = to be taken three times daily; bd = to be taken twice daily; od = to be taken once daily; q4h = to be taken four-hourly.

- Altitude illness   Acetazolamide 250 mg bd (AMS and HACE)
                      Dexamethasone 4 mg qds, oral or iv (HACE and AMS)
                      Nifedipine capsules 10 mg for sublingual use (HAPE)
                      Nifedipine slow release 20 mg tds (HAPE)
                      Oxygen
                      Portable hyperbaric chamber.

* Based on the medical kits used on the following expeditions: British Jaonli Expedition, 1988; British Chamlang Expedition, 1991; British Mount Everest Medical Expedition, 1994.

- Anaesthesia

  Bupivacaine 0.25% (for nerve blocks)
  Ketamine 2 mg/kg over 60 seconds iv (5–10 min of anaesthesia)
  1% lignocaine locally.

- Analgesia

  Anusol (for pruritus ani and haemorrhoids)
  Aspirin 300–600 mg (analgesia, myocardial infarction)
  Codeine phosphate 10–60 mg tds or qds (moderate to severe pain and for diarrhoea)
  Diclofenac 50 mg tds oral/rectal or 75 mg daily im od/bd (anti-inflammatory)
  Naloxone 100–200 micrograms per dose iv
  Opioid analgesic oral/iv/im (e.g. buprenorphine, nalbuphine, for severe pain. Home Office licence recommended for travellers from the UK)
  Paracetamol 1 g q4h (simple analgesic for headaches etc.).

- Asthma and anaphylaxis

  Adrenaline (0.5–1 mg im) (anaphylaxis)
  Becotide/Flixotide metered-dose inhaler
  Chlorpheniramine (10 mg iv) (anaphylaxis)
  Hydrocortisone (100 mg iv) (anaphylaxis)
  Prednisolone 10–20 mg daily
  Salbutamol metered-dose inhaler (asthma, bronchospasm).

- Cardiac

  Aspirin 75 mg daily (myocardial infarct)
  Consider antiarrhythmics
  Frusemide 40 mg iv or oral (congestive cardiac failure)
  Sublingual nitrate (angina).

- Central nervous system

  Chlorpromazine 25–50 mg im or 25 mg tds orally (psychosis, may be induced by dexamethasone)
  Diazepam 5 mg oral/iv (anxiety/sedation)
  Temazepam 10 mg (insomnia).

- Ear and nose

  Chlorpheniramine 4 mg qds or terfenadine 60 mg bd (hayfever)
  Oxymetazoline nasal spray (nasal congestion)
  Steroid nasal spray (allergic rhinitis).

- Eyes

  Amethocaine drops (anaesthesia for examination, emergency evacuation)
  Chloramphenicol ointment (infections and snowblindness)
  1% cyclopentolate (snowblindness)
  Fluorescein
  Sunglasses/goggles (snowblindness).

- Gastrointestinal

  Codeine phosphate 15–30 mg or Lomotil (2–4 tablets and then 2 tablets every 6–8 hours) or loperamide (4 mg and then 2 mg after each loose stool) (diarrhoea)
  Gaviscon/antacid (gastritis)
  Oral rehydration sachets (diarrhoea)
  Prochlorperazine 5 mg tds oral or 12.5 mg im (sublingual is useful for nausea and vomiting)
  Ranitidine 150 mg bd (gastritis/peptic ulcer)
  Senna (constipation).

- Infections

  Amoxycillin/clavulanic acid 500 mg tds (otitis/pneumonia/UTI/skin infections, etc.)
  Ceftriaxone 1–4 g od (penicillin allergic and severe infections)
  Ciprofloxacin 500 mg oral bd (diarrhoea/urinary tract infection)
  Clotrimazole cream (topical fungal infections)
  Cotrimoxazole 480 mg
  Doxycycline 100 mg
  Erythromycin 250 mg qds (atypical pneumonia/penicillin allergy)
  Flucloxacillin 250 mg qds oral or iv (staphylococcal infection)
  Malathion or permethrin (scabies/lice)

Metronidazole 400 mg (*Giardia*/persistent diarrhoea, appendicitis, etc.)
Penicillin 1–5 MU/day iv.

- Malaria   If in malarious areas – antimalarials (prophylaxis and treatment, seek current advice)
Mosquito repellant and nets
Quinine (600 mg tds for one week) and/or mefloquine for treatment.

- Metabolic   Glucagon injection
Insulin (when accompanied by diabetic).

- Oral and throat   Bonjela or Difflam lozenges (sore mouth)
Throat lozenges (sore throat).

- Skin   Calamine lotion/flamazine cream
Chlorpheniramine 4 mg (pruritus)
Factor 15 or higher sunblock
1% hydrocortisone cream (severe sunburn/eczema, etc.)
KY Jelly
White soft paraffin.

- Sterilization and cleaning   Alcohol swabs
Iodine (also for water purification).

Equipment

- Diagnostic equipment   Auriscope
BM Stix
Ophthalmoscope
Pulse oximeter
Spacer for inhaled drugs
Sphygmomanometer
Spirometer (e.g. Micro Medical microspirometer, but not Wright peak flow meter)
Stethoscope
Thermometer (including low-reading).

- Dressings   A variety of dressings
Cotton wool

<table>
<tr><td></td><td>Crepe bandage
Eye pads
Gloves
Penknife with scissors and blade
Steri-strips®
Tape (micropore and elastoplast)
Triangular bandage.</td></tr>
<tr><td>• Intravenous fluids and equipment</td><td>Butterflies
Consider intravenous fluids (Haemacel/saline)
Luer plugs
Needles
Syringes
Take cannulae and giving sets (even if not carrying fluids).</td></tr>
<tr><td>• Surgical and miscellaneous equipment</td><td>Chest drain and Heimlich valve
Consider further surgical equipment depending on expertise, artery forceps, scalpel, scissors, suture holder, craniotomy set!
Consider purpose-made splints
Foley catheter
Nasogastric tube and 50-ml syringe (for aspirating the tube)
Surgical blade
Surgical gloves
Sutures and steri-strips®.</td></tr>
</table>

Injectable drugs checklist

- Adrenaline

- Antiarrhythmic

- Bupivacaine

- Ceftriaxone

- Chlorpheniramine

- Dexamethasone

- Diazepam
- Diclofenac
- Flucloxacillin
- Frusemide
- Glucagon
- Hydrocortisone
- Ketamine
- Lignocaine
- Naloxone
- Opiate
- Penicillin
- Prochlorperazine
- Sodium chloride for injection
- Water for injection.

Personal medical kit (when no doctor is present)

Clear instructions for use of each drug should be included with each kit.

- Acetazolamide
- Codeine phosphate or Lomotil or loperamide
- Diclofenac
- Dressings
- Paracetamol
- Suncream and spare sunglasses
- Throat lozenges.

(On treks, dexamethasone and nifedipine should be carried by the group leader who is familiar with their appropriate use, and by individual climbers on mountaineering expeditions.)

Further reading

A'Court CHD, Stables RH and Travis S (1995) Doctor on a mountaineering expedition. *BMJ*. **310**: 1248–52.

Forgey WW (1995) *Wilderness Medical Society Practice Guidelines for Wilderness Emergency Care*. ICS Books, Merrillville, IN.

Murdoch DR, Pollard AJ and Gibbs S (2001) High altitude and expedition medicine. In: J Zuckerman and A Zuckerman (eds) *Principles and Practice of Travel Medicine*. John Wiley & Sons, Chichester, pp. 247–60.

Appendix 2

The Lake Louise acute mountain sickness scoring system

Several scoring systems have been used to define and quantify AMS in the research setting. Most take the form of self-assessment questionnaires, while others are completed by physicians and include pertinent examination findings. In an attempt to establish a standardized scoring system, the Lake Louise AMS scoring system was developed in 1991. The goal was to create a system with enough sensitivity, specificity and flexibility to allow use in many different settings, that is simple to administer and would enable easier comparisons between studies. This system has since been used by many investigators and has compared well with previous standards. It has therefore been recommended that the Lake Louise AMS scoring system be adopted as the standard for AMS research.

The Lake Louise Score

Self-report questionnaire

1	Headache	0	No headache
		1	Mild headache
		2	Moderate headache
		3	Severe headache, incapacitating.
2	Gastrointestinal symptoms	0	No gastrointestinal symptoms
		1	Poor appetite or nausea
		2	Moderate nausea or vomiting
		3	Severe nausea and vomiting, incapacitating.

3	Fatigue and/or weakness	0	Not tired or weak
		1	Mild fatigue/weakness
		2	Moderate fatigue/weakness
		3	Severe fatigue/weakness, incapacitating.

4	Dizziness/lightheadedness	0	Not dizzy
		1	Mild dizziness
		2	Moderate dizziness
		3	Severe dizziness, incapacitating.

5	Difficulty sleeping	0	Slept as well as usual
		1	Did not sleep as well as usual
		2	Woke many times, poor night's sleep
		3	Could not sleep at all.

Clinical assessment

6	Change in mental status	0	No change in mental status
		1	Lethargy/lassitude
		2	Disoriented/confused
		3	Stupor/semi-consciousness
		4	Coma.

7	Ataxia (heel-to-toe walking)	0	No ataxia
		1	Manoeuvres to maintain balance
		2	Steps off line
		3	Falls down
		4	Can't stand.

8	Peripheral oedema	0	No peripheral oedema
		1	Peripheral oedema at one location
		2	Peripheral oedema at two or more locations.

Functional score

Overall, if you had any symptoms, how did they affect your activity?

0   No reduction in activity
1   Mild reduction in activity
2   Moderate reduction in activity
3   Severe reduction in activity (e.g. bedrest).

The sum of the responses to the questions is calculated, and it is recommended that the scores for the self-report questionnaire, the clinical assessment (if performed) and the functional score be reported separately. A score of three points or greater on the AMS self-report questionnaire alone, or in combination with the clinical assessment score, constitutes AMS.

Given the non-specific nature of symptoms, signs and laboratory findings, there is no 'gold standard' for the diagnosis of AMS. AMS scoring systems, such as the Lake Louise system, are the best available but have shortcomings. In particular, while being relatively sensitive tools, specificity can be variable. Many non-altitude-related conditions may result in a positive diagnosis of AMS.

The diagnosis of acute mountain sickness in preverbal children: The Children's Lake Louise Score (CLLS)

The Lake Louise scoring system for acute mountain sickness is useful in adults but cannot be applied directly to preverbal children (i.e. children under 3 years of age). The Lake Louise scoring system was modified using a fussiness score (FS) as the equivalent to headache, and additional scores for eating (E), playfulness (P) and sleep (S). Fussiness is defined as a state of irritability without a readily identifiable cause, such as hunger, wet nappy (diaper), teething, or pain from an injury or ear infection. Fussiness is scored on a scale of 1 to 6 with regard to amount (duration) and intensity. The sum of both the amount and intensity is equal to FS.

Gastrointestinal complaints are assessed on the basis of the child's appetite and the presence of vomiting (E). Fatigue and weakness questions are replaced by an assessment of the amount of playful activity (P), and the sleep disturbance score applies either to overnight sleep or to sleep during the afternoon napping period (S). The CLLS score is the sum of FS + E + P + S (*see* Figure 1). The CLLS score used to define the presence of AMS must be ≥ 7 with both FS ≥ 4 and E + P + S ≥ 3.

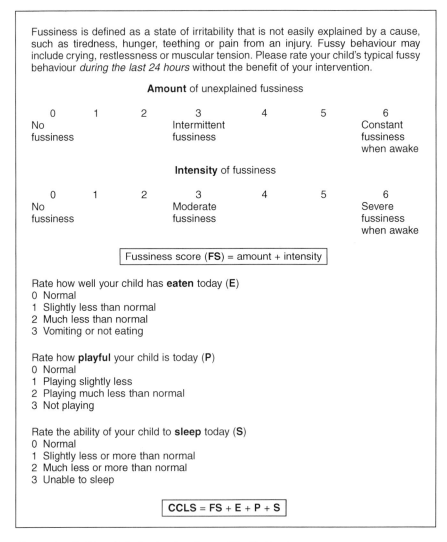

Figure 1: Children's Lake Louise Score (CLLS): fussiness score.

Diagnostic criteria for AMS in the preverbal child should increase awareness of this entity and help clinicians and parents to evaluate a fussy child with appetite, activity and sleep alterations at high altitude. Prompt recognition of AMS in infants may limit their distress and help to prevent dehydration as a result of food refusal or vomiting. The presence of signs beyond those routinely associated with AMS should raise the question of more serious altitude-associated illness (e.g. pulmonary hypertension, pulmonary oedema or other medical conditions).

Further reading

Roach RC, Bärtsch P, Hackett PH *et al.* and the Lake Louise AMS Scoring Consensus Committee (1993) The Lake Louise acute mountain sickness scoring system. In: JR Sutton, CS Houston and G Coates (eds) *Hypoxia and Molecular Medicine*. Queen City Printers, Burlington, VT.

The Lake Louise consensus on the definition and quantification of altitude illness. In: JR Sutton, G Coates and CS Houston (eds) (1992) *Hypoxia and Mountain Medicine*. Queen City Printers, Burlington, VT.

Yaron M, Waldman N, Niermeyer S *et al.* (1998) The diagnosis of acute mountain sickness in pre-verbal children. *Arch Pediatr Adolesc Med.* **152**: 683–7.

Yaron M, Niermeyer S, Lindgren K *et al.* (2002) Evaluation of diagnostic criteria and incidence of acute mountain sickness in preverbal children. *Wild Environ Med.* **13**: 21–6.

Appendix 3

Case histories

AMS

A 24-year-old trekker flew to 2800 m in the Nepal Himalaya and walked for the rest of the day to a village at a similar altitude. His sleep that night was characterized by frequent wakening, and he arose in the morning with a headache that disappeared within an hour. He did not feel like eating breakfast and, once on the trail, found his exercise tolerance was reduced, especially walking uphill. The latter half of the day was spent climbing 600 m up a hillside to a village at 3440 m. During the climb the headache returned and he began to feel nauseated. On reaching the village, all he wanted to do was to go to bed. He had no appetite and needed encouragement from his companion to drink. The next day he still had a headache, but this was much milder. His appetite and exercise tolerance remained poor throughout the day and he spent most of the time resting in his lodge. After a second night at 3440 m, he was almost back to normal. However, he and his companion decided to stay an extra night in the village to acclimatize more fully. He remained well for the rest of their journey, ascending to 5545 m over another six days.

HACE

A 40-year-old male trekker flew to 2800 m and ascended to 3900 m over three days. By the end of the third day he had a headache and felt nauseated. He went to bed without an evening meal. The following morning he felt better, although still had a dull headache. After a normal breakfast he walked slowly on to the next village at 4300 m. He arrived at the village late in the day and went immediately to bed without eating. After a disturbed night, he woke feeling nauseated and with a headache. Despite good advice to the contrary, he insisted that he continue with his plan. He took all day to ascend to the next village at 4700 m, but needed a porter to carry all his gear. That night he vomited and was noted to be very unsteady on his feet. The following morning his porter had difficulty rousing him from sleep and, even when awake, he remained very drowsy and had difficulty standing. Too tired to complain, he was carried down to 3200 m over six hours, where he was seen by a doctor. At this stage his consciousness had improved, but he exhibited marked ataxia on attempting to walk. There was no evidence of HAPE. He was given dexamethasone and two hours' treatment in a portable hyperbaric chamber with further improvement. After an uneventful night, he was able to descend further with assistance. Two days later he caught a scheduled plane and flew to low altitude where he recovered completely. He continued to experience mild ataxia for two days after returning to low altitude.

HAPE

A 22-year-old Nepali soldier, travelling to a new posting, flew from 1300 m to 2800 m and walked to his barracks at 3440 m in one day. That evening, he developed a headache and had difficulty sleeping. The following morning his headache was worse, he had no appetite and felt short of breath on minimal exertion. His condition deteriorated throughout the day such that by evening he was short of breath even at rest. When seen by a doctor he was noted to be cyanosed, had a respiratory rate of 48 per minute and crackles were heard throughout both lung fields. Arterial oxygen saturation by pulse oximetry was 40%. He was given nifedipine and carried that night down to a village at 2800 m. By morning he had improved considerably and had a respiratory rate of 20 per minute at rest. He was sufficiently well two days later to reascend slowly to his barracks at 3440 m. He was advised to ascend more slowly in future.

Appendix 4

Selected elevations

Europe

Elbrus (Russia)	5633 m
Mont Blanc (France/Italy)	4807 m
Monte Rosa (Switzerland/Italy)	4633 m
Matterhorn (Switzerland/Italy)	4478 m
Zermatt (Switzerland)	1616 m
Ben Nevis (Scotland, UK)	1343 m
Snowdon (Wales, UK)	1085 m
Scafell Pike (England, UK)	978 m
Oxford (UK)	60 m

Asia

Mount Everest (Nepal/Tibet)	8848 m
K2 (Pakistan)	8611 m
Kanchenjunga (Nepal/India)	8586 m
Annapurna (Nepal)	8091 m
Thorong La (Nepal)	5400 m
Everest Base Camp (Nepal)	5300 m
Mount Ararat (Turkey)	5185 m
Khunjerah Pass (Pakistan/China)	4709 m
Kinabalu (Malaysia)	4094 m
Mount Fuji (Japan)	3776 m
Lhasa (Tibet)	3658 m
Leh (India)	3514 m

Darjeeling (India)	2127 m
Srinagar (India)	1588 m
Kathmandu (Nepal)	1220 m

Africa

Kilimanjaro (Tanzania)	5895 m
Mount Kenya (Kenya)	5199 m
Mount Cameroon (Cameroon)	4070 m
Pico de Teide (Canary Islands)	3718 m
Addis Ababa (Ethiopia)	2440 m
Johannesburg (South Africa)	1760 m
Nairobi (Kenya)	1660 m

North America

Mount McKinley/Denali (USA)	6194 m
Mount Logan (Canada)	5950 m
Popocatépetl (Mexico)	5452 m
Mount Rainier (USA)	4392 m
Pikes Peak (USA)	4301 m
Leadville (USA)	3100 m
Mexico City (Mexico)	2350 m
Denver (USA)	1610 m

South America

Aconcagua (Argentina)	6959 m
Huascarán (Peru)	6768 m
Cerro de Pasco (Peru)	4265 m
Potosi (Bolivia)	3960 m
La Paz (Bolivia)	3625 m
Cuzco (Peru)	3415 m
Quito (Ecuador)	2850 m
Bogota (Colombia)	2640 m

Oceania/Pacific

Carstensz Pyramid (Indonesia)	5030 m
Mount Wilhelm (Papua New Guinea)	4509 m
Mauna Kea (Hawaii)	4205 m
Mount Cook/Aoraki (New Zealand)	3754 m
Mount Kosciusko (Australia)	2228 m
Christchurch (New Zealand)	8 m

Antarctica

Vinson Massif	5140 m
South Pole	3000 m

Appendix 5

Height, pressure and temperature conversion table

Metres	Feet	Pressure (mmHg)	Approximate temperature (°C)	(°F)
0	0	760	15	59
1000	3281	674	8.5	47.3
2000	6562	596	2	35.6
3000	9843	526	−4.5	23.9
4000	13 123	463	−11	12.2
5000	16 404	405	−17.5	0.5
6000	19 685	354	−24	−11.2
7000	22 966	308	−30.5	−22.9
8000	26 247	267	−37	−34.6
8848	29 029	236	−42	−43.6

Appendix 6

Fact sheet for altitude illness (adapted with permission from a draft document prepared by David Hillebrandt)

AMS is a serious medical condition that can quickly lead to HACE and/or HAPE which are life-threatening emergencies. Any signs or symptoms should be reported to the expedition leader or doctor.

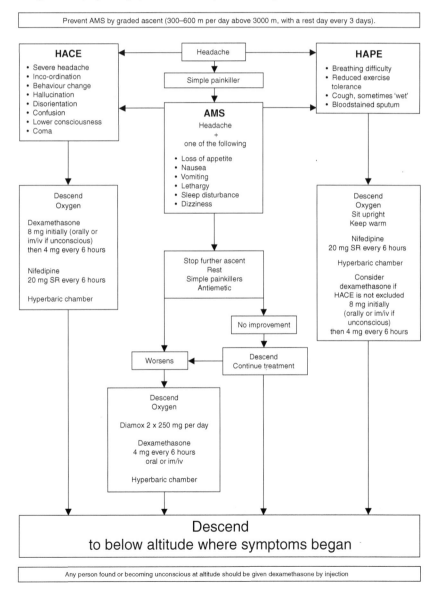

Prevent AMS by graded ascent (300–600 m per day above 3000 m, with a rest day every 3 days).

HACE
- Severe headache
- Inco-ordination
- Behaviour change
- Hallucination
- Disorientation
- Confusion
- Lower consciousness
- Coma

Headache

Simple painkiller

AMS
Headache
+
one of the following
- Loss of appetite
- Nausea
- Vomiting
- Lethargy
- Sleep disturbance
- Dizziness

HAPE
- Breathing difficulty
- Reduced exercise tolerance
- Cough, sometimes 'wet'
- Bloodstained sputum

Descend
Oxygen

Dexamethasone
8 mg initially (orally or im/iv if unconscious) then 4 mg every 6 hours

Nifedipine
20 mg SR every 6 hours

Hyperbaric chamber

Stop further ascent
Rest
Simple painkillers
Antiemetic

No improvement

Worsens

Descend
Continue treatment

Descend
Oxygen

Diamox 2 x 250 mg per day

Dexamethasone
4 mg every 6 hours
oral or im/iv

Hyperbaric chamber

Descend
Oxygen
Sit upright
Keep warm

Nifedipine
20 mg SR every 6 hours

Hyperbaric chamber

Consider dexamethasone if HACE is not excluded
8 mg initially (orally or im/iv if unconscious) then 4 mg every 6 hours

Descend
to below altitude where symptoms began

Any person found or becoming unconscious at altitude should be given dexamethasone by injection

Appendix 7

Fact sheet for doctors: prevention and treatment of altitude illness

Prevention

Acute mountain sickness

1 Gradual ascent – e.g. average 300–600 m/day with rest day every 1000 m or every 3 days.
2 Drug prophylaxis:
   - Acetazolamide
     - 250 mg bd (or 500 mg slow-release nocte) from at least 24 hours prior to ascent above 2500 m
     - lower doses, e.g. 125 mg bd, are under investigation
   - Dexamethasone
     - 4 mg every 6–8 hours from at least 24 hours prior to ascent above 2500 m
     - usually only used by those intolerant of or allergic to acetazolamide.

High altitude pulmonary oedema

1 As for acute mountain sickness.
2 Nifedipine, e.g. 20 mg slow-release every 8 hours, can be considered for those with a known susceptibility to HAPE.

High altitude cerebral oedema

1 As for acute mountain sickness.

Treatment

Acute mountain sickness

Mild
1 Rest (stop further ascent)
2 Simple analgesia/antiemetics as required.

Moderate/severe
1 Descent
2 Oxygen
3 Acetazolamide 250 mg tds
4 Dexamethasone 4 mg qds
5 Hyperbaric chamber.

High altitude pulmonary oedema

1 Descent
2 Sit upright
3 Oxygen
4 Nifedipine 20 mg slow-release qds
5 Hyperbaric chamber.

High altitude cerebral oedema

1 Descent
2 Oxygen
3 Dexamethasone 8 mg, then 4 mg every 6 hours
4 Hyperbaric chamber.

Appendix 8

Useful addresses and telephone numbers

Mountaineering organizations

Alpine Club, 55/56 Charlotte Road, London EC2A 3QF, UK. Tel: 020 7613 0755. Website: http://www.alpine-club.org.uk

The Alpine Club of Canada, PO Box 8040, Indian Flats Road, Canmore, Alberta, Canada T1W 2T8. Tel: 403 678 3200. Website: http://www.alpineclubofcanada.ca/

American Alpine Club, 710 Tenth Street, Golden, CO 80401, USA. Tel: +1 303 384 0110. Website: http://www.americanalpineclub.org

Australian Sport Climbing Federation, PO Box 1043, Artarmon, NSW 1570, Australia. Tel: 0418 248 804. Fax: 02 9818 7118. Website: http://www.climbing.com.au/ascf/ascf.htm

British Mountaineering Council (BMC), 177–179 Burton Road, West Didsbury, Manchester M20 2BB, UK. Tel: 0870 010 4878. Fax: 0161 445 4500. Website: http://www.thebmc.co.uk. The BMC runs mountaineering courses and can offer advice about other courses which are approved by them and about insurance.

Deutscher Alpenverein, Hauptgeschaeftsstelle, von Kahr-Str 2–4, 80997 Muenchen, Germany or Postfach 50 0220, 80972 Muenchen, Germany. Tel: +49 89 140030. Fax: +49 89 1400311. Website: http://www.alpenverein.de

Expedition Advisory Centre of the Royal Geographical Society, 1 Kensington Gore, London SW7 2AR, UK. Tel: 020 7591 3030. Fax: 020 7591 3031. Website: http://www.rgs.org

The New Zealand Alpine Club, PO Box 786, Christchurch, New Zealand. Website: http://www.nzalpine.org.nz/

Austrian Alpine Club (UK branch), PO Box 43, Welwyn Garden City, Herts AL8 6PT, UK. Tel: 01707 386 740. Website: http://www.aacuk.uk.com/

Japanese Alpine Club, 5-4 Yonban-cho Chiyoda-ku, Tokyo 102-0081, Japan. Tel: +81 3 3261 4433. Fax: +81 3 3261 4441. Website: http://www.jac.or.jp

Club Alpino Italiano. Website: http://213.140.0.212:8080/index.jsp

Club Alpin Français d'Ile-de-France, 12 rue Boissonade, 75014 Paris, France. Website: http://www.clubalpin-idf.com/

The Scottish Mountaineering Club. Website: http://www.smc.org.uk/

Schweizerischer Alpenclub, Geschaeftsstelle Monbijou Str 61, CH 3000, Bern. Tel: +41 31 370 1818. Fax: +41 31 370 1800. Website: http://www.sac-cas.ch

The Ski Club of Great Britain, The White House, 57–63 Church Road, Wimbledon, London SW19 5SB, UK. Tel: 0845 45 807 80. Fax: 0845 45 807 81. Website: http://www.skiclub.co.uk/

Travel medicine advice

Address for Home Office drug licence application: Room 239, Drugs Branch, Home Office, 50 Queen Anne's Gate, London SW1H 9AT, UK. Tel: 020 7273 3806. Email: licensing_enquiry.aadu@homeoffice.gsi.gov.uk Website: http://www.homeoffice.gov.uk/atoz/drugs.htm

Centers for Disease Control and Prevention. Website: http://www.cdc.gov/

Medical Advisory Services for Travellers Abroad. Website: http://www.masta.org/

Travel Health online. Website: http://www.tripprep.com/

International Travel and Health (World Health Organization). Website: http://www.who.int/ith/

Health Canada Travel Medicine Program. Website: http://www.hc-sc.gc.ca/pphb-dgspsp/tmp-pmv/

Health Advice for Travellers, Department of Health, UK. Website: http://www.doh.gov.uk/traveladvice/

University College London Hospital (UCLH) Hospital for Tropical Diseases Travel Clinic. Travellers Healthline Advisory Service. Tel: 09061 33 77 33. Website: http://www.uclh.org/services/htd/travelclinic.shtml

Malaria prevention guidelines. Website: http://www.malaria-reference.co.uk/

Malaria advice for doctors: Tel: 0121 766 6611 (Birmingham)
01865 225217 (Oxford)
020 7636 3924 (London, Malaria Reference Laboratory, prophylaxis only)
020 7387 4411 (Hospital for Tropical Diseases, London)
0906 708 8807 (School of Tropical Diseases, Liverpool)
0141 300 1130 (Glasgow)

Malaria advice for the public: Email: health.services@britishairways.com
09065 508908 (Malaria Reference Laboratory, Public Health Laboratory Service).

Recorded advice for travellers. Tel: 0891 600350.

Wilderness medicine, mountain rescue medicine and high altitude medicine websites

Avalanche Emergency Homepage: http://www.provinz.bz.it/avalanche

Bibliography of High Altitude Medicine and Physiology. Website: http://annie.cv.nrao.edu/habibqbe.htm

Birmingham Medical Research Expeditionary Society. Website: http://www.bmres.org.uk/

CIWEC Clinic, Travel Medicine Center, Kathmandu, Nepal. Website: http://ciwec-clinic.com/

Deutsche Gesellschaft für Berg- und Expeditionsmedizin (BExMed) e.V. Website: http://www.lrz-muenchen.de/~bexmed/

Himalaya Rescue Association. Website: http://www.himalayanrescue.com

Institut d'Estudis de Medicína de Muntanya (IEMM). Website: http://www.iemm.org/

International Commission for Mountain Rescue. Website: http://www1.vrz.net/public/ikar-cisa.nsf/Design/HTML/FramesetHomepage

International Porter Protection Group. Website: http://www.ippg.net/

International Society for Mountain Medicine. Website: http://www.ismmed.org

International Society of Travel Medicine. Website: http://www.istm.org/

Medex and Medical Expeditions. Website: http://www.medex.org.uk/

Mountain Medicine and Traumatology Department of Chamonix Hospital (DMTM). Website: http://perso.wanadoo.fr/dmtmcham/dmtm_uk.htm

Österreichische Gesellschaft für Alpin- und Höhenmedizin. Website: http://www.alpinmedizin.org

Schweizerischen Gesellschaft für Gebirgsmedizin. Website: http://www.mountainmedicine.ch/

UIAA Mountain Medicine Centre. Website: http://www.thebmc.co.uk/world/mm/mm0.htm

UIAA (Union Internationale des Associations d'Alpinisme/The International Mountaineering and Climbing Federation). Website: http://www.uiaa.ch/

Wilderness Medical Society. Website: http://www.wms.org

Further reading

Auerbach P (ed.) (2001) *Wilderness Medicine. Management of wilderness and environmental emergencies* (4e). Mosby, St Louis, MO.

Bezruchka S (1994) *Altitude Illness: prevention and treatment*. Cordee, Leicester.

Bollen S (1989) *First Aid on Mountains*. British Mountaineering Council, Manchester.

Forgey WW (ed.) (2000) *Wilderness Medical Society Practice Guidelines for Wilderness Emergency Care* (2e). Globe Pequot, Guilford, CT.

Heath D and Williams DR (1995) *High Altitude Medicine and Pathology* (4e). Oxford University Press, Oxford.

Hornbein TF and Schoene RB (eds) (2001) *High Altitude: an exploration of human adaptation. Lung Biology in Health and Disease, Volume 161*. Marcel Dekker, New York.

Houston C (1998) *Going Higher: man, oxygen and mountains*. The Mountaineers, Seattle, WA.

Hultgren H (1997) *High Altitude Medicine*. Hultgren Publications, Stanford, CA.

Reeves JT and Grover RF (eds) (2001) *Attitudes on Altitude: Pioneers of Medical Research in Colorado's High Mountains*. University of Colorado Press, Boulder, CO.

Steedman DJ (1994) *Environmental Medical Emergencies*. Oxford University Press, Oxford.

Steele P (1999) *Medical Handbook for Walkers and Climbers*. Constable, London.

Vallotton J and Dubas F (1991) *A Colour Atlas of Mountain Medicine*. Wolfe, London.

Ward MP, Milledge JS and West JB (2000) *High Altitude Medicine and Physiology* (3e). Edward Arnold, London.

Wilkerson J (ed.) (2001) *Medicine for Mountaineering and Other Wilderness Activities* (5e). Mountaineers Books, Seattle, WA.

Selected journals

High Altitude Medicine and Biology is published by Mary Ann Liebert Inc. Website: http://www.liebertpub.com/HAM/default1.asp

Journal of Travel Medicine is published by BC Decker. Website: http://www.istm.org

Wilderness and Environmental Medicine is published by the Wilderness Medical Society. Website: http://www.wemjournal.org/wmsonline

Glossary

Acclimatization – the process of physiological adjustment to the lack of oxygen following arrival at a new altitude.

Acute mountain sickness (AMS) – the milder, more common form of altitude illness characterized by symptoms of headache, nausea, vomiting, loss of appetite, poor sleep and lethargy.

Adaptation – the process of physiological adjustment to lack of oxygen at high altitudes that occurs over decades to generations.

Aetiology – the cause of a disease.

Amaurosis fugax – sudden loss of vision.

AMS – *see* acute mountain sickness.

Analgesia – relief of pain.

Anorexia – loss of appetite.

Antiemetics – medicines which stop vomiting.

Anti-platelet agents – medicines which reduce the stickiness of platelets and the risk of unwanted blood clotting.

Aorta – the major blood vessel which takes blood from the heart to the rest of the body.

Apnoea – cessation of breathing – respiratory arrest.

Asystole – cessation of heartbeat – cardiac arrest.

Ataxia – inco-ordination, clumsy movement (e.g. the stumbling unsteady walk seen in HACE).

Auscultation – listening with a stethoscope.

bd – twice daily.

Bitemporal hemianopia – partial blindness with loss of vision at the sides.

Bradycardia – slowness of heart rate.

Bronchospasm – reversible narrowing of the airways caused by contraction of smooth muscle in the walls of the air passages.

Bullae – large fluid-filled blisters on damaged skin.

Capillary – small blood vessel.

Carapace – a hard covering of stiff dead tissue.

Carbonic anhydrase – an enzyme which converts carbon dioxide and water into carbonic acid (a weak acid).

Cardiological review – review by a heart specialist.

Carotid artery – large blood vessel in the neck supplying blood to the brain.

Cerebral – of the brain.

Cerebrovascular accident – stroke.

Chemoprophylaxis – preventative medication.

Cholecystitis – inflammation of the gall-bladder.

Clubbing – abnormal curving of the fingernails, associated with certain heart and lung diseases.

Coma – unconscious state.

Conjunctiva – the delicate membrane lining the eyelids and covering the eyeball.

Contralateral – opposite side.

Core temperature – temperature measured in the mouth or rectum.

Cornea – transparent covering over the pupil of the eye.

Cortical blindness – blindness caused by damage to the part of the brain involved in seeing, rather than by an abnormality of the eye.

Coryza – discharge from the nose, as occurs with a 'common cold'.

Cranial nerves – the 12 nerves supplying the muscles and sensory organs of the head and neck, which arise directly from the brain rather than from the spinal cord.

Cyanosis – blue coloration of the skin and mucosa caused by a reduction in the amount of oxygen carried by the blood.

Cycloplegic – causes dilation of the pupil and paralysis of the ciliary muscle.

Debridement – surgical removal of dead tissue (e.g. skin).

Denervated – relating to a tissue such as skin or muscle which has lost its nerve supply (e.g. numb skin).

Desaturation – reduction in the amount of oxygen in the blood ('oxygen saturation').

Diuresis – increased production of urine.

Diverticulitis – inflammation of a diverticulum.

Diverticulum – a pouch or sac protruding from the bowel wall.

Doppler echocardiography – a technique which allows the blood flow in the heart and large blood vessels to be measured with an ultrasound machine.
Ductus arteriosus – a small blood vessel which connects the main lung artery to the main body artery (aorta); it normally closes soon after birth.
Dysphasia – difficulty in speaking because of an abnormality in the brain, such as a stroke.
Dyspnoea – laboured or difficult breathing.
Ectopic – 'in the wrong place' (e.g. an embryo growing outside the womb instead of in the womb).
Electively – 'not as an emergency'.
Electrolyte – an ionic salt (dissolved in the blood) such as sodium, potassium or calcium.
Enteral – via the gut (e.g. by mouth).
Epidemiology – the study of the distribution of diseases within a population.
Epistaxis – nosebleed.
Erythropoietin – a substance that stimulates the production of red blood cells.
Ex-prems – babies born prematurely who have survived the newborn period.
Extracellular fluid – fluid which bathes the tissues of the body.
Extracorporeal – 'outside the body'.
Gastrocolic reflex – contraction of the colon after stimulation of the stomach with food.
Gastrointestinal disturbance – abdominal upset such as diarrhoea, vomiting or abdominal pain.
Glucagon – a hormone which increases the amount of glucose in the blood.
HACE – *see* high altitude cerebral oedema.
Haematemesis – vomiting blood.
Haematocrit – the volume of red blood cells relative to the total volume of fluid in the blood.
Haemoglobin – the molecule which carries oxygen in the blood.
Haemorrhages – areas of bleeding.
HAPE – *see* high altitude pulmonary oedema.
Heimlich valve – a valve which allows air to be drained out of the chest without allowing air back in.
Hemianopia – *see* bitemporal hemianopia.
Hemiparesis – paralysis of one side of the body.

Hepatomegaly – enlargement of the liver.

High altitude cerebral oedema (HACE) – a serious form of altitude illness in which excess fluid accumulates in the brain.

High altitude pulmonary oedema (HAPE) – a serious form of altitude illness in which excess fluid accumulates in the lungs.

Hyperaemia – increased blood flow causing a red coloration.

Hyperbaric – high environmental pressure.

Hyperbilirubinaemia – the presence in the blood of high levels of the pigment bilirubin, which is normally removed by the liver.

Hypercapnia – high levels of carbon dioxide in the blood.

Hyperhidrosis – excessive sweating.

Hypernatraemia – high blood sodium levels.

Hyperpnoea – increased rate of breathing.

Hypersensitivity – increased sensitivity.

Hyperviscosity – excessive thickness of a liquid.

Hypnotic – an agent that induces sleep.

Hypobaric – low environmental pressure.

Hypocapnia – deficiency of carbon dioxide in the blood.

Hypoglycaemia – low levels of glucose in the blood.

Hyponatraemia – low levels of sodium in the blood.

Hypotension – low blood pressure.

Hypothermia – low body temperature.

Hypovolaemia – low blood volume (e.g. caused by bleeding or dehydration).

Hypoxaemia – low levels of oxygen in the blood.

Hypoxia – low levels of oxygen.

Infarction – interruption of the blood supply, causing tissue death.

Intercostal – between the ribs.

Intra-ocular – inside the eye.

Intravenous – into the veins.

Ischaemia – a critical reduction in blood supply.

Ketoacidosis – a life-threatening condition that affects diabetics with dehydration and high blood glucose levels.

Lavage – 'washing out' of a body cavity with sterile fluid.

Macula – part of the back of the eye involved in central vision.

Malabsorption – failure to absorb food in the gut, often resulting in diarrhoea and weight loss.

Mandible – lower jaw and jaw joint.

Menarche – onset of menstruation (periods) during puberty.

Mucosa – the body tissue covering the surfaces of the mouth, windpipe, food pipe, airways and gut.

Myalgia – muscle pain.

Myocardial infarct – heart attack.

Nasogastric tube – a tube that is inserted into the stomach via the nose to enable delivery of medicines or fluid into the gut.

Neonate – a baby from birth to one month of age.

Nerve palsy – paralysis of a part of the body caused by nerve damage.

Neurological examination – examination of the body to look specifically for signs of injury to the nerves, spinal cord or brain.

Normothermic – normal temperature.

Occipital – the back of the head (over the part of the brain involved with sight).

od – once daily.

Oedema/oedematous – swelling of a tissue.

Oliguria – production of abnormally small quantities of urine.

Oral – by mouth.

Oximeter – a device which uses absorbance of red light to measure the amount of oxygen in the blood.

Oxygen saturation – the amount of oxygen in the blood, measured by an oximeter.

Paediatrics – the study of children's medicine.

Pancreatitis – inflammation of the pancreas.

Paraesthesia – numbness, tingling and altered sensation.

Paralytic ileus – loss of normal contractions of the bowel.

Parenterally – administration of a drug or fluid by a means other than via the gut (e.g. intravenously).

Pathogenesis – the mechanism that occurs in the development of disease.

Pathophysiology – the physiological processes involved in the development of disease.

Peptic ulcer – a stomach ulcer.

Perineum – the area of skin between the legs around the genitals.

Peritoneum – the lining of the walls of the abdomen and pelvis.

Petechial – small areas of bleeding in the skin or some other organ.

Pneumothorax – an air leak around the lung (usually) caused by an injury to the chest which potentially compromises the ability to breathe.

po – by mouth.

Polycythaemia – an increase in the number of red blood cells in the bloodstream (in response to lack of oxygen at altitude).

Post-mortem – autopsy.

Prophylaxis – preventive treatment.

Pulmonary – 'of the lung'.

qds – four times a day.

Raynaud's syndrome – a disease in which the blood supply to the fingers is affected, usually in response to cold exposure, resulting in white numb fingers.

REM – a phase of sleep known as rapid eye movement sleep.

Respiratory depression – a reduction in the drive to breathing.

Retina – the area at the back of the eye which detects light.

Reye's syndrome – a severe illness that affects children, associated with the use of aspirin.

Rhinorrhoea – runny nose.

Salpingitis – inflammation of the Fallopian tubes.

Saturation – *see* oxygen saturation.

Scotomata – loss of part of the field of vision.

Sickle-cell disease – an inherited blood disorder in which the red blood cells are more fragile than normal, and when stressed take up a sickle shape.

Snowblindness – solar damage (sunburn) to the outer surfaces of the eye.

Somnolence – sleepiness.

Spirometer – a device for measuring lung function.

Sputum – phlegm.

Subclinical – without overt symptoms.

Sublingual – under the tongue.

Syncope – a faint.

Tachycardia – fast heart rate.

Tachypnoea – fast breathing rate.

tds – three times a day.

Tendinitis – inflammation of tendons.

Thrombosis – blood clot.

Transient ischaemic attack – a stroke-like episode with paralysis or loss of function, which recovers completely.

Valsalva's manoeuvre – a technique that consists of closing the mouth and nose and blowing, which forces the pressure inside the chest cavity to increase.

Vasoconstriction – narrowing of blood vessels brought about by muscle contraction in the walls of those blood vessels.

Vasodilation – widening of blood vessels brought about by relaxation of the muscles in their walls.

Vasodilator – a medicine which dilates blood vessels.

Vasospastic – spasm of blood vessels, leading to a reduction in the flow of blood.

Venesection – 'taking of blood from a blood vessel'.

Ventilatory – breathing.

Ventricular fibrillation – unco-ordinated contraction of the heart muscles so that no pumping action is possible.

Vestibular apparatus – the part of the inner ear which detects movement and orientation and thus balance sensation.

Vestibular sedatives – medicines which suppress the sensation of motion, used to treat motion sickness.

Viscus – an organ such as the liver, spleen, etc.

Zygomatic arch – cheekbone.

Index